Geriatrics

Editor

PAUL RAITI

VETERINARY CLINICS OF NORTH AMERICA: EXOTIC ANIMAL PRACTICE

www.vetexotic.theclinics.com

Consulting Editor
JÖRG MAYER

September 2020 • Volume 23 • Number 3

ELSEVIER

1600 John F. Kennedy Boulevard • Suite 1800 • Philadelphia, Pennsylvania, 19103-2899
http://www.vetexotic.theclinics.com

VETERINARY CLINICS OF NORTH AMERICA: EXOTIC ANIMAL PRACTICE Volume 23, Number 3
September 2020 ISSN 1094-9194, ISBN-13: 978-0-323-72085-4

Editor: Stacy Eastman
Developmental Editor: Nicole Congleton

Veterinary Clinics of North America: Exotic Animal Practice (ISSN 1094-9194) is published in January, May, and September by Elsevier, Inc., 360 Park Avenue South, New York, NY 10010-1710. Subscription prices are $287.00 per year for US individuals, $545.00 per year for US institutions, $100.00 per year for US students and residents, $338.00 per year for Canadian individuals, $657.00 per year for Canadian institutions, $352.00 per year for international individuals, $657.00 per year for international institutions, $100.00 per year Canadian students/residents, and $165.00 per year for international students/residents. To receive student/resident rate, orders must be accompanied by name of affiliated institution, date of term, and the *signature* of program/residency coordinator on institution letterhead. Orders will be billed at individual rate until proof of status is received. Foreign air speed delivery is included in all *Clinics* subscription prices. All prices are subject to change without notice. **POSTMASTER:** Send address changes to *Veterinary Clinics of North America: Exotic Animal Practice*, Elsevier Health Sciences Division, Subscription Customer Service, 3251 Riverport Lane, Maryland Heights, MO 63043. **Customer Service: Telephone: 1-800-654-2452** (U.S. and Canada); **1-314-447-8871** (outside U.S. and Canada). **Fax: 1-314-447-8029. E-mail: journalscustomerservice-usa@elsevier.com (for print support); journalsonlinesupport-usa@elsevier.com (for online support)**.

Reprints. For copies of 100 or more of articles in this publication, please contact the Commercial Reprints Department, Elsevier Inc., 360 Park Avenue South, New York, New York 10010-1710. Tel.: 212-633-3874; Fax: 212-633-3820; E-mail: reprints@elsevier.com.

Veterinary Clinics of North America: Exotic Animal Practice is covered in *MEDLINE/PubMed (Index Medicus)*.

Contributors

CONSULTING EDITOR

JÖRG MAYER, Dr med vet, MSc
Diplomate, American Board of Veterinary Practitioners (Exotic Companion Mammals); Diplomate, European College of Zoological Medicine (Small Mammals); Diplomate, American College of Zoological Medicine; Associate Professor of Zoological Medicine, Department of Small Animal Medicine and Surgery, University of Georgia College of Veterinary Medicine, Athens, Georgia, USA

EDITOR

PAUL RAITI, DVM
Diplomate of the American Board of Veterinary Practitioners (Reptile and Amphibian Practice); Beverlie Animal Hospital, Mount Vernon, New York, USA

AUTHORS

TERESA BRADLEY BAYS, DVM, CVA, CVMMP
Diplomate American Board of Veterinary Practitioners (Exotic Companion Mammals); Belton Animal Clinic and Exotic Care Center, Belton, Missouri, USA

SHANE BOYLAN, DVM
Chief Veterinarian, South Carolina Aquarium, Charleston, South Carolina, USA

JOHN CHITTY, BVetMed, CertZooMed, MRCVS
Anton Vets, Hants, United Kingdom

MICHAEL DUTTON, DVM, MS
Diplomate, American Board of Veterinary Practitioners (Canine & Feline Practice); Diplomate, American Board of Veterinary Practitioners (Avian Practice); Diplomate, American Board of Veterinary Practitioners (Exotic Companion Mammal Practice); Diplomate, American Board of Veterinary Practitioners (Reptile & Amphibian Practice); Exotic and Bird Clinic of New England, c/o Weare Animal Hospital, Weare, New Hampshire, USA

DENISE M. IMAI, DVM, PhD
Diplomate, American College of Veterinary Pathologists; Comparative Pathology Laboratory, University of California, Davis, California, USA

DAN H. JOHNSON, DVM
Diplomate, American Board of Veterinary Practitioners (Exotic Companion Mammal); Avian and Exotic Animal Care, Raleigh, North Carolina, USA

CATHY A. JOHNSON-DELANEY, DVM
Special Projects, NW Zoological Supply, Everett, Washington, USA

BENJAMIN KENNEDY, MSc, BVetMed, MRCVS, Mem RES
Anton Vets, Anton Trading Estate, Andover, United Kingdom

ANGELA M. LENNOX, DVM
Diplomate, American Board of Veterinary Practitioners (Avian, Exotic Companion Mammal); Diplomate, European College of Zoological Medicine (Small Mammal); Avian and Exotic Animal Clinic, Indianapolis, Indiana, USA

MICHELLE O'BRIEN, BVetMed, CertZooMed, MRCVS
Diplomate, European College of Zoological Medicine (Zoo Health Management); Wildfowl & Wetlands Trust, Gloucester, United Kingdom

SARAH PELLETT, BSc(Hons), MA, VetMB, CertAVP(ZM), MRCVS
Diploma in Zoological Medicine(Reptilian); Animates Veterinary Clinic, Thurlby, Lincolnshire, United Kingdom

DRURY R. REAVILL, DVM
Diplomate, American Board of Veterinary Practitioners (Avian and Reptile & Amphibian Practice); Diplomate, American College of Veterinary Pathologists; ZNLabs Veterinary Diagnostics, Citrus Heights, California, USA

TITUS FRANCISCUS SCHEELINGS, BVSc, MVSc, PhD, MANZCVSc (Wildlife Health)
Diplomate, European College of Zoological Medicine (Herpetology); Alphington, Victoria, Australia

Contents

> As pain management finally becomes accepted for this last of the verte-
> brate taxa, fish medicine is finally reaching the sophistication of other ver-
> tebrates. The diseases of aging fish in captivity therefore need to be
> addressed. The degenerative organ/tissue changes and neoplasias of
> fish deserve the same diagnosis and treatments of their terrestrial counter-
> parts including pain relief, anti-inflammatory medications, chemotherapy,
> surgery, joint supplements, regenerative cell therapy, and photobiomodu-
> lation. Besides the challenges of an aquatic environment, recognizing
> normal changes in older fish will be addressed in this article. Clinicians
> can appreciate the diversity of fishes and their unique anatomies, physiol-
> ogies, and behaviors which translate to creative medicine.

> Captive amphibians and reptiles may be extraordinarily long-lived pets,
> with some species able to reach ages of more than 150 years. Therefore,
> such longevity needs to be contemplated before purchasing an animal.
> Similar to traditional companion species, the health and husbandry re-
> quirements of herpetofauna change throughout the course of their lives,
> and modifications to how animals are kept need to take this into consider-
> ation. Regular examinations, including diagnostics, are invaluable in moni-
> toring the health of senescent amphibians and reptiles and may aid in
> assessing quality of life.

> Despite falconry having been practiced for centuries and with a wealth of
> published material on the husbandry of captive raptors over that period,
> there is a paucity of published material on the care of the geriatric raptor.
> Raptors are often a long-lived species and can suffer a range of age-
> related conditions that may impact on their welfare. This article seeks to
> cover some of these conditions and look at welfare considerations in the
> management of geriatric raptors, including quality-of-life assessments
> and euthanasia decision making.

African hedgehogs are susceptible to aging changes like those of other small exotic mammals. Common conditions of the geriatric hedgehog include heart disease, chronic renal disease, and dental/periodontal disease. Hedgehogs are unique in that they have an unusually short life span and a propensity for neoplasia. These 2 factors make it especially common for exotic animal practitioners to encounter geriatric hedgehogs affected by one of the many conditions outlined in this article.

A great deal of attention has been directed toward developing better options for palliative care and hospice, and improving euthanasia techniques in all species. Euthanasia of exotic pets is technically more difficult because of anatomic differences and small patient size. Traditional intravenous euthanasia techniques in conscious patients are stressful and should generally be avoided in exotic pets; simple intramuscular administration of high dosages of anesthetics followed by delivery of euthanasia solutions is preferred. Options for mammals, birds, and reptiles are presented.

The review covers select disease conditions most frequently described in aging rodents (rats, mice, hamsters, guinea pigs), rabbits, and ferrets. The conditions are categorized by general organ systems, infectious diseases, and neoplasms. Two data systems, the Veterinary Medical Teaching Hospital and Comparative Pathology Laboratory at the University of California, Davis and Zoo/Exotic Pathology Service, Citrus Heights, California were used in the determining disease conditions to describe.

Supplement article:

VETERINARY CLINICS OF NORTH AMERICA: EXOTIC ANIMAL PRACTICE

SERIES OF RELATED INTEREST

Veterinary Clinics of North America: Small Animal Practice
Available at: https://www.vetsmall.theclinics.com/

THE CLINICS ARE NOW AVAILABLE ONLINE!
Access your subscription at:
www.theclinics.com

Preface

Geriatrics Issue 2020

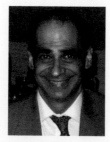

Paul Raiti, DVM, DABVP (Reptile and Amphibian Practice)
Editor

This publication provides a continuation and advancement of pertinent information (ie, therapeutics) regarding geriatric management of "exotic" pets, including fish (freshwater and marine), reptiles, amphibians, psittacines, raptors, rats, mice, hamsters, gerbils, ferrets, rabbits, guinea pigs, chinchillas, hedgehogs, and invertebrates. The current issue will be more fully appreciated when paired with the original *Veterinary Clinics of North America: Exotic Animal Practice* Geriatrics Issue of 2010 to which mice, hamsters, gerbils, chinchillas, hedgehogs, and invertebrates have currently been added. Additional articles for 2020 include Palliative Care, Hospice, and Euthanasia (A. Lennox) and Pathology of Diseases of Geriatric Exotic Mammals (D. Reavill and D. Imai-Leonard). The mammalian pathology article complements the article on Pathology of Geriatric Psittacines (D. Reavill and G. Dorrestein) in the 2010 issue. M. Bercier's article on psittacines is available on the Veterinary Clinics: Exotic Animal Practice website, https://www.vetexotic.theclinics.com/. As longevity has generally increased for "exotic" pets, quality-of-life issues and veterinary support have moved more to the forefront for management of these pets. A mentor of mine repeatedly said that the veterinarian's responsibility is "not always to cure but always to care," and this has been a personal goal throughout my veterinary career. Being a clinician, I asked each author to emphasize the use of pictures as a teaching aid, and all generously responded, which I thank them for. Please enjoy and learn from the following pages.

Paul Raiti, DVM, DABVP (Reptile and Amphibian Practice)
Beverlie Animal Hospital
Mount Vernon, NY 10552, USA

E-mail address:
praiti1@verizon.net

Vet Clin Exot Anim 23 (2020) ix
https://doi.org/10.1016/j.cvex.2020.06.001
1094-9194/20/© 2020 Published by Elsevier Inc.

Geriatric Freshwater and Marine Fish

Shane Boylan, DVM

KEYWORDS

- Medicine • Teleost • Elasmobranch • Geriatrics • Radiography

KEY POINTS

- Veterinarians should be aware that as fish age, significant changes can occur to gender, swim bladders, and skeletal structures that are normal. Recognizing what is normal and what is pathology is critical.
- The same diseases that affect older terrestrial vertebrates affect fish like vertebral disk disease, neoplasia, and uroliths. Treatments should include regenerative medicine, anti-inflammatories, nutritional supplements, surgery, chemotherapy, photobiomodulation, and pain control.
- Diagnostics like ultrasound, endoscopy, radiography, computed tomography, and magnetic resonance imaging are invaluable assets in fish medicine. Their use is informative and should be utilized as the aquatic environment is not an impediment to imaging when done properly.

Fish medicine should still be considered in its infancy, as fish represent the last vertebral taxa that still does not have 100% consensus on whether they feel pain. It should be no surprise then that geriatric fish medicine is rarely discussed as a separate topic. "Geriatric" is an adjective that relates to the health care of "the old." Geriatric fish medicine may mean recognizing normal age changes and not attributing those changes as pathology. We often do not know the life expectancy of most fishes (plurality of multiple fish species) in the wild, and we cannot anticipate how the benefits of captivity prolong their longevity. Greenland sharks have been found to be the longest-lived vertebrates on our planet with an expected longevity of 400 years and average life spans of 272 years. Growth curves suggest female Greenland sharks reach sexual maturity at 156 years of age.[1] Big Mouth Buffalo (*Ictiobus cyprinellus*) have the oldest estimated longevity for freshwater teleosts (most ray-finned fishes) at 112 years.[2] In captivity, some fish may double their life expectancy when predation and food scarcity are removed as mortality factors. What we hope to do as fish clinicians is improve the quality of life and expand our understanding with each species.

The lack of veterinary fish knowledge can overwhelm the new clinician, but abundant information can be found in the fisheries literature if the clinician has the time to

South Carolina Aquarium, 100 Aquarium Wharf, Charleston, SC 29401, USA
E-mail address: sboylan@scaquarium.org

Vet Clin Exot Anim 23 (2020) 471–484
https://doi.org/10.1016/j.cvex.2020.05.001
1094-9194/20/© 2020 Elsevier Inc. All rights reserved.

search. This article presents some of the normal and abnormal changes that fish experience as they age because these life histories are not part of the normal veterinary education. Fishes outnumber all the other vertebrate taxa with approximately 33,400 species (fishbase.org), which is more than the sum of the other taxa: amphibians, reptiles, birds, and mammals. The diversity among fishes cannot be overstated. Although elasmobranchs (sharks, rays, skates) and teleosts are similar in their use of fins and gills, their anatomic and physiologic similarities end there. Most veterinarians would be concerned with blood urea nitrogen values in the 700 to 2000 mg/dL, yet that is normal for many elasmobranchs, which use urea nitrogen as part of their buoyancy control. Elasmobranchs lack swim bladders, true bone, and the ribs present in most, but not all, teleosts. Elasmobranchs use an epigonadal organ and not the head kidney of teleosts for primary hematopoiesis. The elasmobranch rectal gland does much of sodium/chloride regulation of the teleost gill. Several texts are now available on fish medicine that include descriptions of the unique physiologies and environmental parameters that veterinarians need to know to be effective clinicians.[3–8]

Neoplasia is a common complication in geriatric fish. The fish literature and Registry of the Tumor of Lower Animals contains numerous examples of fish neoplasia.[9,10] Despite public perception, neoplasia also occurs in elasmobranchs, although perhaps less frequently then in their teleost cousins.[11–13] Soft tissue sarcoma and myxosarcomas are common histopathological diagnoses of koi coelomic masses. Most of these neoplasias are not metastatic, although they can be locally infiltrative. Treatment is often excisional with surgical steel or radiosurgery. Superficial masses can be removed with scalpel excision followed by liquid nitrogen cryotherapy, which may reduce recurrence.[14] Chemotherapy attempts have been published, and clinicians should be encouraged to add more modalities to neoplasia treatment beyond simple excision.[15] An excellent synopsis of fish oncology is published.[9]

The discussion of fish geriatrics is system based. The primary focus of this discussion of geriatrics involves ornamental and public aquaria fishes. Aquaculture species are represented in this article typically through reports of neoplasia usually associated with brood stock. It should be noted that all treatments mentioned are not approved by the Food and Drug Administration for fish intended for human consumption. Geriatric medicine for fish is the same for geriatric medicine for other vertebrates. Joint supplements, regenerative medicine, cold laser therapy, and anti-inflammatory medications should all be considered.

MUSCULOSKELETAL SYSTEM

The support of the aquatic environment may explain the lack of geriatric orthopedic issues in fish. Spinal issues, especially spondylosis, may be the most common age-related finding, and factors like tanks design, nutrition, trauma, and handling are likely to be significant contributing factors.[16,17] Veterinarians are very familiar with spondylosis and intervertebral disk disease among certain canine breeds with long backs like dachshunds. Vertebrae that lack ribs also lack the support of intercostal ligaments, and these vertebrae are more susceptible to degenerative changes during aging. A variety of large fish (elasmobranchs, moray eels) possess no ribs, and it is no surprise that these fishes represent the "aquatic dachshunds" in fish medicine. Handling of these fishes out of water requires complete body support to avoid vertebral trauma. Sedation is suggested, as struggling, long-bodied fishes may injure their own back and injure their handlers, especially when they are removed from the support of water. Sandtiger sharks (*Carcharias taurus*) suffer vertebral disease at all ages from issues

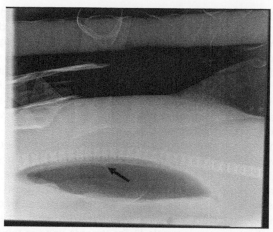

Fig. 1. Antemortem, lateral view of a juvenile sandtiger shark (*Carcharias taurus*) radiograph through a stretcher showing a suspected vertebral issue (*arrow*) highlighted by negative contrast effect of air in the stomach, which is normal for sandtigers.

related to tank design/swimming pattern, handling-related trauma, and potential nutritional deficiencies.[18] Although age is not known to be a major contributor to sandtiger scoliosis, any evaluation of an older sandtiger shark should consider vertebral health as part of the examination. Sandtiger scoliosis is a progressive, degenerative disease. In the author's experience, most sandtiger sharks' clinical symptoms progress over months to years. The sharks continue to eat despite becoming hunched and twisted with kyphosis and scoliosis, respectively. Sandtigers have tolerated repeat injections of dexamethasone (0.5–1.0 mg/kg intramuscularly [IM]), oral prednisolone (1–2 mg/kg orally [PO]), and glycoaminoglycans (Adequan), although there is no way to evaluate if they had any benefit. In one instance, the author radiographed 3 young sandtigers through their stretchers that supported them on their move from quarantine to display

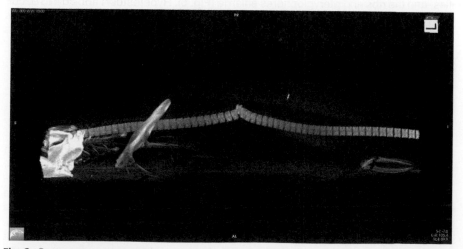

Fig. 2. Postmortem computed tomography (CT) maximal intensity projection (MIP) of same juvenile sandtiger (*Carcharias taurus*) from **Fig. 1** with pronounced vertebral disk disease.

tanks. One of the 3 animals displayed a spinal anomaly (**Fig. 1**) that presented as kyphosis 6 months after imaging. This shark's clinical symptoms dramatically progressed during 3 weeks, and it was euthanized. Postmortem analysis showing significant vertebral spondylosis with ventral cartilage proliferation that is common among sandtiger sharks that experienced years of degeneration (**Fig. 2**). Although this case is not an example of geriatric disease, the rapid progression of lesions should be considered possible in older sandtiger sharks. Vitamins E, C, and selenium supplementation may be preventive, and handling of animals should always proceed with care with this species, especially in reproductive females and geriatric animals.

A report of spondylosis in an adult green moray eel revealed degenerative notocord/disklike material with corresponding radiographic findings of compressed intervertebral disk spaces.[16] Clinical symptoms of reduced mobility, failure to control swim bladder volume, and inappetance correspond to nerve damage in the areas of the vertebral compression. Steroids produced minimal benefits, and cold laser therapy appeared to alleviate vertebral-associated symptoms, just as it assists with vertebral osteoarthritis complications in mammals.[16] Treatments used in mammals should be considered in geriatric spinal disease of fish, including pain medication (gabapentin, opioids), stem cell therapy, joint supplements, vertebroplasty, photobiomodulation, and acupuncture whenever possible. Trauma-caused spinal damage often occurs from collisions with tank walls/structures. Although not directly caused by age, older fish have more chances to suffer trauma, just as older koi in outdoor ponds have increased risk of spinal damage from lightning strikes because they have lived longer. Necropsy radiographs have often found incidental, old, healed spinal injuries that the fish carried throughout their life without clinical symptoms. Thus, geriatric fish should have their spines imaged whenever possible so pain management and supplements can be used to improve quality of life (**Figs. 3** and **4**).

Hyperostosis is an adult-onset condition that is normal for many saltwater species of teleosts. Expansion of bone in the ribs, pterygiophores, hemal spines, and neural bones can easily be mistaken for mammalian hyperostosis caused by hypervitaminosis D or hyperfluorosis. **Fig. 5** demonstrates the normal skeleton of a young Atlantic spadefish where the supra occipital bone is not calcified, and all ribs, neural bones, and pterygiophores appear normal. As this species ages, the supraoccipital crest calcifies, and the ribs and pterygiophores enlarge (**Fig. 6**). Hyperostosis appears to occur

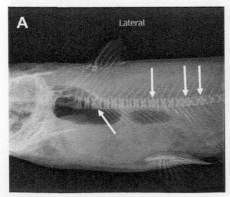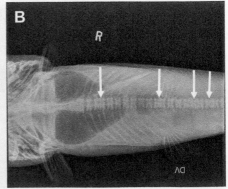

Fig. 3. (*A, B*) Antemortem lateral and dorsal-ventral radiographs of a geriatric channel catfish (*Ictalurus punctatus*) with spinal compression (*arrows*).

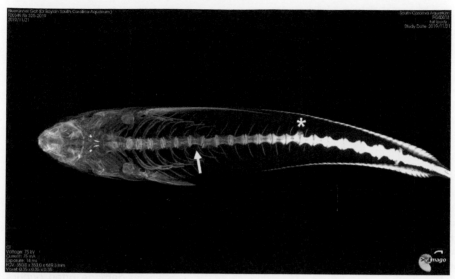

Fig. 4. Postmortem geriatric blue runner (*Caranx crysos*) post-CT MIP revealing scoliosis (*arrow*) and disk rupture (*asterisk*).

most commonly among marine eels and fish in the Carangidae family. An excellent publication is available that summarizes the condition.[19]

Neoplasia in the fish musculoskeletal system is going to occur more commonly in older fish. Numerous tumors are reported, including osteomas and rhabdomyosarcomas.[20]

OCULAR

Cataracts are a common phenomenon in aquaria and aquaculture. Nutrition and parasitism are common causes of cataracts in aquaculture. Age is a factor in

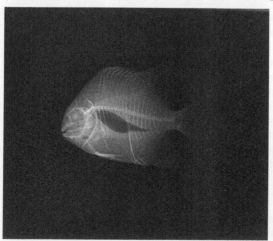

Fig. 5. Antemortem juvenile Atlantic spadefish (*Chaetodon faber*) lateral radiograph revealing normal skeleton and swim bladder. The supraoccipital crest is uncalcified and all ribs, neural bones, and pterigophores have normal shape. The swim bladder is consistent among teleost fish except for a caudal extension.

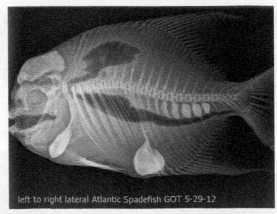

left to right lateral Atlantic Spadefish GOT 5-29-12

Fig. 6. Adult Atlantic spadefish (*Chaetodon faber*) lateral radiograph with calcification of the supra-occipital crest and hyperostosis of ribs, and pterigophores. The swim bladder has bifurcated both cranially and caudally. Cranial swim bladder protrusions proceed dorsal to vertebral column.

cataract occurrence in public aquaria and pet fish, but the lack of predation and prevalence of food often compensates for reduced vision. In acute cases, phaco-emulsification can be very successful in restoring vision. Most chronic eye injuries result in lens avulsion, which can be treated by making an incision into the cornea and removing the displaced lens with forceps (lensectomy). In these chronic cases, the retina is often destroyed, but it should be noted that fish experience retinal growth as they age, so regeneration is more possible than with their terrestrial vertebrate counterparts.

Lipid keratopathy is a dietary and perhaps age-related condition among moray eels. Eel captive diets likely have higher fat content, either through high-fat food items or increased feeding frequency. When combined with age, several eel species develop lipid corneal deposition that obstructs vision. Dietary correction and removal of affected spectacles were successful in improving vision.[21]

Adipose lids are precursors to traditional palpebrae. These static, periocular structures support the eye during swimming by reducing hydrostatic forces. Adipose lids may change in clarity during reproduction by deposition of lipids. As fish age and undergo repeated reproduction, the adipose lids appear to lose their clarity. Older Carangidae fish (family of ray-finned fish that includes the jacks, pompanos, jack mackerels, runners, and scads) tend to accumulate adipose lid tissue, which can cover and obscure the eyes. Hypertrophy of adipose lids has been documented in scad, although new evidence suggests the phenomenon appears to be more related to water temperature than age.[22] Surgical excision and cryotherapy may be palliative in geriatric fish with excessive adipose lid accumulation.

SWIM BLADDER

Clinicians need to recognize that the swim bladder is a dynamic organ. The swim bladder participates in hearing, communication, and buoyancy, and it should be no surprise that the shape and function of swim bladders changes as fish age. Drumming fish use their swim bladder to communicate during reproduction, and therefore their swim bladders change significantly as they sexually mature. As red drum (*Scianaeops ocellatus*) grow, their swim bladder develops lateral projections that use special

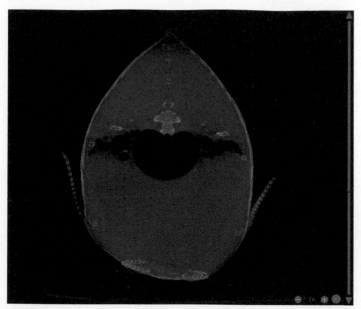

Fig. 7. Transverse CT section of a red drum, *Sciaenops ocellatus*, swim bladder revealing the lateral projections that participate in drumming.

muscles to drum during breeding season. Imaging of the swim bladder projections could be interpreted as pathology if the life history of the fish is unknown (**Fig. 7**). Similarly, Atlantic spadefish, *Chaetodon faber*, demonstrate some of the most dynamic change in swim bladders among any marine teleost. In juvenile to sub-adult spadefish

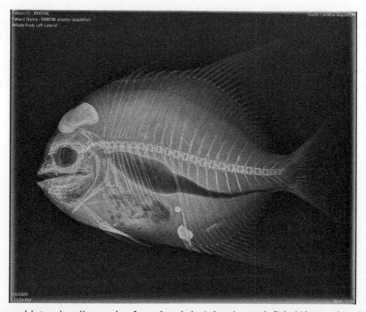

Fig. 8. Normal lateral radiograph of a sub-adult Atlantic spadefish (*Chaetodon faber*).

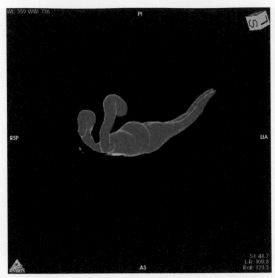

Fig. 9. Three-dimensional reconstruction from a CT of an adult Atlantic spadefish (*Chaetodon faber*) swim bladder showing the asymmetric shaped cranial projections.

(**Fig. 8**), the "classic" swim bladder is present except for a caudal tapering. As the spadefish age, the swim bladder generates 2, asymmetric cranial projections that proceed dorsal to the vertebral column during maturity (**Fig. 9**). Caudally, the swim bladder also bifurcates into 2 projections that extend to the last caudal vertebrae. The adult swim bladder shape becomes dorsal-ventrally compressed compared with a juvenile, presumably to compensate for the changes in total gas volume as the swim bladder elongates cranially and caudally. The asymmetric cranial projections likely facilitate in sound detection like the asymmetric ears in owls. As with red drum, these changes occur in adulthood and contribute to the reproductive strategies of these fishes. Clinicians need to understand these changes are normal, and that older fish often have the most significant changes.

Spondylosis, which is more common in geriatric fish, may alter innervation to the swim bladder, which can alter its normal function. Sympathetic and parasympathetic

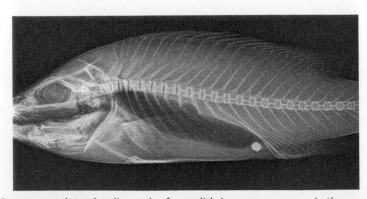

Fig. 10. Postmortem lateral radiograph of a urolith in a gray snapper, *Lutjanus griseus*.

innervation from the spinal cord controls gas secretion and absorption as demonstrated in studies severing or antagonizing nerves that altered the return to volume of deflated swim bladders.[23,24] Older fish with spinal disease may experience swim bladder inflation abnormalities, which was suspected in a case in a moray eel.[16]

Swim bladder–associated neoplasia is uncommon, but a gas gland adenoma has been reported in a sea horse and a swim bladder fibrosarcoma in Atlantic salmon.[25,26] Coelomic masses, often of ovarian or testicular origin, can compress or invade the swim bladder.[27]

UROGENITAL SYSTEM

Uroliths are an uncommon finding among fish. Their presence in the absence of inflammation suggest many uroliths are incidental findings on necropsy and postmortem imaging (**Fig. 10**). Renal disease is rarely diagnosed antemortem among fishes. Teleost gills and elasmobranch rectal glands do much of the electrolyte balancing normally attributed to mammalian kidneys. The anemia associated with mammalian renal disease does not commonly occur in fish. The erythropoietin secreted by mammalian kidneys is an evolutionary connection to fish anatomy when the hematopoietic head and tail kidneys fused. Although anemia is a common complaint in fish, clinicians should rule out prerenal causes like poor water quality or infectious disease (proliferative kidney disease for example) before jumping to primary renal disease. The best example of piscine primary kidney disease occurs in geriatric sandtigers who often die with primary renal failure (Robert George, personal communication, 2017).

Renal tubular neoplasia has been documented in an oscar and a nephroblastoma in smelt.[28,29] Reproductive tumors are commonly reported in both teleosts and

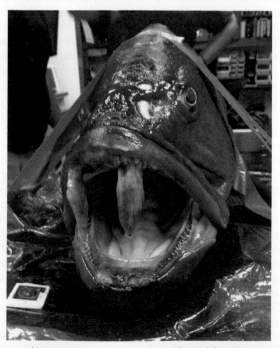

Fig. 11. A gag grouper (*Mycteroperca microlepis*) with proliferative oral epithelium associated with age.

elasmobranchs.[30–32] Given that the gills, rectal glands, and the gastrointestinal system assist with functions normally associated with mammalian kidneys, it should be no surprise that most renal neoplasias are difficult to diagnose with bloodwork and instead are identified by antemortem imaging of coelomic swellings or necropsy.

OROPHARYNGEAL AND GASTROINTESTINAL SYSTEM

A common geriatric condition among captive fishes in the snapper grouper complex is the proliferation of the dorsal oral epithelial tissue (**Fig. 11**). Geriatric grouper/snappers are prone to hypertrophy of the oral epithelium, which can be described as hairlike stalactites that can be seen when they open their mouths. The etiology could be related to a papilloma/retro virus or a lack of normal "wear and tear" in the mouth. It is a cosmetic issue, and the author has trimmed this tissue with scissors and used liquid nitrogen cryotherapy to successfully prevent recurrence.

Another common complaint in predatory geriatric fishes is the inability to close the mouth. The complex jaw protrusion mechanism of predatory fish likely suffers from age-related joint disease. These fish survive in captivity if they learn to seine food into the rear of the pharynx. On examination, the mouth can be closed with pressure, but the jaws spring open once released. In the author's experience, muscle relaxers (1 mg/kg midazolam IM) minimally alleviate the symptoms in the short term, and computed tomography imaging has failed to identify any joint that would explain the condition. If a traumatized or dislocated joint could be identified, the condition may be corrected similar to treatment in human temporomandibular syndrome. If the etiology is related to a tendon or ligament, surgery may be able to alleviate the symptoms.

Oral neoplasias with papillomalike characteristics have been reported in wild blue sharks, captive sandtiger sharks, wild great white sharks, and catfish.[12,33,34] In teleosts, odontomas in barracuda and sarcomas in the jaws of needlefish are described.[35,36] Fibromas with a possible viral etiology have been found on the lips of angelfish.[37] Superficial oral masses can be treated with excision and cryotherapy.

Enteroliths are even more rare than uroliths. An enterolith has been reported in sandtiger sharks, and the author has found an enterolith in a nurse shark.[38]

LIVER AND GALL BLADDER

Hepatic lipidosis is one of the most common findings in geriatric fish. It should not be assumed to be as pathologic in fish as it is in mammals. Wild-caught predatory fish often have lipid-rich livers. Most carnivorous fish are fed to satiation in captivity to reduce predation, and many of these species store lipid in the liver compared with coelomic fat. For this reason, most sharks and teleosts like lionfish have significant hepatic lipid stores. Fish with excess hepatic lipid may suffer more lipid peroxidation during inappetence, but there is scant evidence to compare the condition with mammals. Ultrasound is an excellent way to evaluate the liver in geriatric fish, and dietary supplements like s-adenosyl methionine and silybin may be warranted with severe hepatic lipidosis. Cholelithiasis is rare in fish, but biliary disease can be detected by ultrasound in species with gall bladders and possibly treated with ursodiol when surgery is unwarranted (Robert George, personal communication). Clinicians should be aware that many shark species, like nurse sharks (*Ginglymostoma cirratum*), lack gall bladders (Boylan, personal observation).

Hepatic neoplasia is common in toxin/carcinogen-exposed zebrafish, and spontaneous hepatoblastomas and hepatic cholangiocarcinoma have been reported in elasmobranchs and teleosts.[31,39,40]

ENDOCRINE

Goiter is a common disease in captivity, and it should be addressed in geriatrics, as iodine deficiency is more likely to occur in adults. Ozone and high nitrates reduce the bioavailability of sea water iodine, which is normally abundant.[41,42] Most marine fishes lack the ability to store iodine or increase the absorption across the gills or intestines when faced with deficiency related to captive conditions. Oral supplementation of potassium iodine 30 mg/kg PO once weekly has been effective for the author in treating geriatric black sea bass (*Centropristis striata*) and blue angelfish (*Holochanthus bermudaensis*) that exhibit seasonal goiter symptoms including masses at the base of the gills and increased gilling rate. The same dosing regimen has effectively treated elasmobranchs with goiter, although chronic conditions rarely totally resolve the gular-associated swellings (Boylan, personal observation). Currently, most multivitamins designed for elasmobranchs use iodate salts, which may not be as effective as potassium iodine. This author uses both a general multivitamin (dose per manufacturer) and potassium iodine to prevent goiter in geriatric elasmobranchs.

INTEGUMENT

Chronic ulcerations are common complaints in geriatric fish. Elasmobranchs are particularly prone to tank wall abrasions, as they often ride tank walls or rub against tank structures. Modifying the tank flow, decreasing population density, and adding barriers are often necessary to prevent recurrence. Topical applications of various creams, powders, and ointments have been beneficial: silver sulfadiazine, silver collocate, becaplermin, and misoprostol-phenytoin combinations. Hole in the head lateral line erosions and atypical mycobacteria should be ruled out with chronic dermal lesions.

Older fish often have excessive skin on their operculums. This change is not pathogenic, but it makes a live, geriatric fish easy to identify. Aging fish usually require postmortem analysis of otoliths, as radiographic density of otoliths does not predict age (Boylan, personal observation).

Dermal neoplasias are uncommon and can be treated with surgical excision, intralesional chemotherapy, and cryotherapy.[9,14,26,43,44]

SUMMARY

Fish can be treated with the same level of sophistication and compassion as all other animals. Many of the same conditions that affect older mammals afflict fish. Perhaps the most difficult issue in geriatric fish medicine is recognizing normal, which was touched on here. Clinicians should see the aquatic environment as a benefit and use it to their advantage to provide their patients with the best quality of life.

DISCLOSURE

No financial conflicts of interest.

REFERENCES

1. Nielsen J, Hedeholm RB, Heinemeier J, et al. Eye lens radiocarbon reveals centuries of longevity in the Greenland shark (*Somniosus microcephalus*). Science 2016;353(6300):702–4.

2. Lackmann AR, Andrews AH, Butler MG, et al. Bigmouth Buffalo *Ictiobus cyprinellus* sets freshwater teleost record as improved age analysis reveals centenarian longevity. Commun Biol 2019;2(1):197.

3. Smith SA, editor. Fish diseases and medicine. Boca Raton (FL): CRC Press; 2019.

4. Stoskopf MK. Fish medicine. Philadelphia: W. B. Saunders Company; 1993.

5. Noga EJ. Fish disease: diagnosis and treatment. John Wiley & Sons; 2010.

6. Saint-Erne N. Advanced Koi care: for veterinarians and professional Koi keepers. Glendale (AZ): Erne Enterprises; 2002.

7. Roberts HE, editor. Fundamentals of ornamental fish health. Ames, Iowa: John Wiley & Sons; 2011.

8. Smith M, Warmolts D, Thoney D, et al. The elasmobranch husbandry manual: captive care of sharks, rays and their relatives. Columbus (OH): Special Publication of the Ohio Biological Survey; 2004.

9. Vergneau-Grosset C, Nadeau ME, Groff JM. Fish oncology: diseases, diagnostics, and therapeutics. Vet Clin Exot Anim Pract 2017;20(1):21–56.

10. Reavill D. Neoplasia in fish. In: Roberts HE, editor. Fundamentals of ornamental fish health. Ames Iowa: Wiley-Blackwell; 2010. p. 204–13.

11. Garner MM. A retrospective study of disease in elasmobranchs. Vet Pathol 2013; 50(3):377–89.

12. Huveneers C, Klebe S, Fox A, et al. First histological examination of a neoplastic lesion from a free-swimming white shark, *Carcharodon carcharias* L. J Fish Dis 2016;39(10):1269–73.

13. Manire CA, Clare AC, Wert D, et al. Lymphosarcoma in a captive bonnethead shark. *Sphyrna tiburo* (L.). J Fish Dis 2013;36(4):437–40.

14. Boylan SM, Camus A, Waltzek T, et al. Liquid nitrogen cryotherapy for fibromas in tarpon, *Megalops atlanticus*, Valenciennes 1847, and neoplasia in lined sea horse, *Hippocampus erectus*, Perry 1810. J Fish Dis 2015;38(7):681–5.

15. Stevens BN, Vergneau-Grosset C, Rodriguez CO Jr, et al. Treatment of a facial myxoma in a goldfish (*Carassius auratus*) with intralesional bleomycin chemotherapy and radiation therapy. J Exot Pet Med 2017;26(4):283–9.

16. Boylan SM, Camus A, Gaskins J, et al. Spondylosis in a green moray eel, *Gymnothorax funebris* (Ranzani 1839), with swim bladder hyperinflation. J Fish Dis 2017;40(7):963–9.

17. Lester RJ, Kelly WR. Ankylosing spondylosis in the giant perch, *Lates calcarifer* (Bloch). J Fish Dis 1984;7(3):193–7.

18. Preziosi R, Gridelli S, Borghetti P, et al. Spinal deformity in a sandtiger shark, *Carcharias taurus* Rafinesque: a clinical–pathological study. J Fish Dis 2006; 29(1):49–60.

19. Smith-Vaniz WF, Kaufman LS, Glowacki J. Species-specific patterns of hyperostosis in marine teleost fishes. Mar Biol 1995;121(4):573–80.

20. Iwanowicz LR, Goodwin AE, Harshbarger JC. Embryonal rhabdomyosarcoma of the giant gourami, *Colisa fasciata* (Bloch & Schneider). J Fish Dis 2001;24(3): 177–80.

21. Clode AB, Harms C, Fatzinger MH, et al. Identification and management of ocular lipid deposition in association with hyperlipidaemia in captive moray eels, *Gymnothorax funebris* Ranzani, *Gymnothorax moringa* (Cuvier) and *Muraena retifera* Goode and Bean. J Fish Dis 2012;35(9):683–93.

22. Boylan SM, Harms CA, Waltzek T, et al. Clinical report: hyperplastic adipose lids in mackerel scad, *Decapterus macarellus* (Cuvier). J Fish Dis 2011;34(12):921–5.

23. Fänge R, Holmgren S, Nilsson S. Autonomic nerve control of the swimbladder of the goldsinny wrasse, *Ctenolabrus rupestris*. Acta Physiol Scand 1976;97(3): 292–303.

24. Finney JL, Robertson GN, McGee CA, et al. Structure and autonomic innervation of the swim bladder in the zebrafish (*Danio rerio*). J Comp Neurol 2006;495(5): 587–606.

25. Duncan IB. Evidence for an oncovirus in swimbladder fibrosarcoma of Atlantic salmon *Salmo salar* L. J Fish Dis 1978;1(1):127–31.

26. Stilwell JM, Boylan SM, Howard S, et al. Gas gland adenoma in a lined seahorse, *Hippocampus erectus*, Perry 1810. J Fish Dis 2018;41(1):171–4.

27. Lewis S, Pinkerton ME, Churgin SM, et al. Abnormal Buoyancy in a Convict Cichlid (*Amatitlania Nigrofasciata*) Associated with an ovarian carcinoma invading the swim bladder. J Exot Pet Med 2016;25(2):106–9.

28. Petervary N, Gillette DM, Lewbart GA, et al. A spontaneous neoplasm of the renal collecting ducts in an oscar, *Astronotus ocellatus* (Cuvier), with comments on similar cases in this species. J Fish Dis 1996;19(4):279–81.

29. Huizinga HW, Budd J. Nephroblastoma in the smelt, *Osmerus mordax* (Mitchill). J Fish Dis 1983;6(4):389–91.

30. Masahito P, Ishikawa T, Takayama S. Spontaneous spermatocytic seminoma in African lungfish, *Protopterus aethiopicus* (Heckel). J Fish Dis 1984;7(2):169–72.

31. Borucinska JD, Harshbarger JC, Bogicevic T. Hepatic cholangiocarcinoma and testicular mesothelioma in a wild-caught blue shark, *Prionace glauca* (L.). J Fish Dis 2003;26(1):43–9.

32. Jafarey YS, Berlinski RA, Hanley CS, et al. Presumptive dysgerminoma in an orange-spot freshwater stingray (*Potamotrygon motoro*). J Zoo Wildl Med 2015; 46(2):382–5.

33. Borucinska JD, Harshbarger JC, Reimschuessel R, et al. Gingival neoplasms in a captive sand tiger shark, *Carcharias taurus* (Rafinesque), and a wild-caught blue shark, *Prionace glauca* (L.). J Fish Dis 2004;27(3):185–91.

34. Poulet F, Wolfe M, Spitsbergen J. Naturally occurring orocutaneous papillomas and carcinomas of brown bullheads (*Ictalurus nebulosus*) in New York State. Vet Pathol 1994;31:8–18.

35. Vijayakumar R, Gopalakrishnan A, Raja K, et al. Occurrence of tumour (odontoma) in marine fish *Sphyraena jello* from the southeast coast of India. Dis Aquat Organ 2014;108(1):53–60.

36. Kiryu Y, Landsberg JH, Bakenhaster MD, et al. Putative histiocytic sarcoma in redfin needlefish *Strongylura notata* (Beloniformes: Belonidae) in Florida, USA. Dis Aquat Organ 2018;132(1):57–78.

37. Francis-Floyd R, Bolon B, Fraser W, et al. Lip fibromas associated with retrovirus-like particles in angel fish. J Am Vet Med Assoc 1993;202(3):427–9.

38. Monreal-Pawlowsky T, Thornton SM, Stidworthy MF, et al. Coeliotomy under general anaesthesia and removal of an enterolith from a sand tiger shark (*Carcharias taurus*). Vet Rec Case Rep 2016;4(2):e000357.

39. Stilwell JM, Camus AC, Zachariah TT, et al. Disseminated lymphoid neoplasia and hepatoblastoma in an Atlantic stingray, *Hypanus sabinus* (Lesueur 1824). J Fish Dis 2019;42(2):319–23.

40. Vogelbein WK, Fournie JW, Cooper PS, et al. Hepatoblastomas in the mummichog, *Fundulus heteroclitus* (L.), from a creosote-contaminated environment: a histologic, ultrastructural and immunohistochemical study. J Fish Dis 1999; 22(6):419–31.

41. Morris AL, Stremme DW, Sheppard BJ, et al. The onset of goiter in several species of sharks following the addition of ozone to a touch pool. J Zoo Wildl Med 2012;1:621–4.
42. Sherrill J, Whitaker BR, Wong GT. Effects of ozonation on the speciation of dissolved iodine in artificial seawater. J Zoo Wildl Med 2004;35(3):347–56.
43. Vorbach BS, Peiffer LB, Clayton LA, et al. Multiple recurrent cutaneous masses in a cownose ray (*Rhinoptera bonasus*) with progression from benign lesions to high-grade carcinoma. J Fish Dis 2019;42(11):1623–7.
44. Wildgoose WH. Papilloma and squamous cell carcinoma in koi carp (*Cyprinus carpio*). Vet Rec 1992;130:153–7.

Geriatric Reptiles and Amphibians

Titus Franciscus Scheelings, BVSc, MVSc, PhD, MANZCVSc (Wildlife Health), DECZM (Herpetology)

KEYWORDS

- Reptiles • Amphibians • Geriatric • Aging • Senescence • Quality of life

KEY POINTS

- Longevity of amphibians and reptiles varies considerably between species, but some are extraordinarily long-lived, necessitating significant commitment from owners.
- Management of geriatric disease in amphibians and reptiles also entails careful consideration of current husbandry practices and may require changes to enclosure design in order to accommodate frail individuals.
- Quality-of-life assessments can be difficult in amphibians and reptiles, but regular examination and reassessment may be invaluable in categorizing and monitoring senescence in individuals.

INTRODUCTION

The emergence of the tetrapod groups Amphibia and Reptilia represented monumental leaps in Earth's biological history. The earliest amphibians evolved from sarcopterygian fish and began to haul themselves from the primordial Devonian swamps (360 million years ago), in order to escape the stagnant, oxygen poor waters.[1] These first vertebrate terrestrial colonists discovered a world devoid of major competition but bursting with opportunity as the floral and invertebrate faunal diversity exploded exponentially. The teleologic advantage of being a terrestrial vertebrate, combined with the smorgasbord of abundant prey items, meant that amphibians could rapidly spread to occupy the vast array of previously vacant ecological niches on offer. However, ultimately, their dominance of the new world was stifled by their reliance on freshwater for reproduction, and it was not until the age of reptiles (Carboniferous period 320 million years ago) that true global supremacy was possible. The defining feature of reptiles that enabled them to displace the amphibians was the advent of the amniotic egg.[2] This marvel of evolution severed the tie that vertebrates had to their aquatic origins and facilitated their rise to the chief life forms on the planet for the next 160 million years.

2/2-10 Fulham Road, Alphington, Victoria 3078, Australia
E-mail address: fscheelings@hotmail.com
Twitter: @fswildvet (T.F.S.)

Vet Clin Exot Anim 23 (2020) 485–502
https://doi.org/10.1016/j.cvex.2020.05.004
1094-9194/20/© 2020 Elsevier Inc. All rights reserved.

Today, it is estimated that there are more than 8000 living species of amphibians[3] and more than 10,000 living species of reptiles.[4] The diversity in form and function of the extant herpetofauna is mind boggling, with some persisting unchanged since their first appearance an eon ago. Despite the physiologic constraints of ectothermy, both reptiles and amphibians have radiated globally and can be found on every continent with the exception of Antarctica.[3,4] Nonetheless, their grip on continued existence is tenuous, as reptiles and amphibians are among the most imperiled species on the planet. It has been shown that nearly 40% of the known amphibian species in existence are at immediate risk of extinction,[3] whereas around 20% of the described reptilian species are threatened with extinction, with another 20% classified as Data Deficient.[5]

Since the dawn of human consciousness, both reptiles and amphibians have occupied a unique place in our history. They are used as an important source of nourishment, and they pervade the fables and stories of almost every human culture, as both villains and heroes. It is perhaps a combination of the role that they have played in shaping the human psyche, their unique appearance and physiology, and their unbroken lineage to an ancient and mysterious world that has so endeared herpetofauna to many pet owners, making them one of the fastest growing pet industries in the United States.[6] With this increase in popularity of amphibians and reptiles as pets comes a concurrent expectation that they receive the same standard of care as traditional companion animals. Consequently, herptile husbandry and medicine has evolved at such a pace that many captive specimens now live far beyond the natural lifespans of their wild counterparts. This subsequent longevity has meant that veterinarians must be aware of the medical conditions associated with geriatric reptiles and amphibians and be adequately equipped to deal with the challenges of elder medicine and end-of-life strategies.

The phylogenetic history of the herpetofauna is complex and is frequently debated with some disagreement on the relatedness of specific taxonomic clades. Although it is still unknown if the Lissamphibia (modern amphibians), represent a monophyletic (share a common ancestor) or paraphyletic (do not share a common ancestor) group,[7] what is generally agreed is that the Reptilia are paraphyletic in their origins.[8,9] This means that adequately encapsulating the life history traits of all species within these groups is difficult, as there is such variety between individuals, even within genera. However, in the context of this article, broad generalizations are possible, in order to give the clinician an overview of senescence in reptiles and amphibians and to outline some of the common medical conditions associated with advanced age in these taxa.

REPRODUCTION, GROWTH, AND AGING IN AMPHIBIANS

Amphibians have complex life cycles with one of the defining features being a dramatic shift in habitat, facilitated by ontogenetic changes in an individual's morphology, physiology, and behavior.[10] For most of the amphibians, fertilization is external, and they are oviparous.[11] However, there are examples of species in which ovoviviparity and viviparity with internal fertilization exist.[12,13] Larvae are usually free-living and aquatic in their habits and through the process of metamorphosis transform physically to their adult form, where they are most often terrestrial and highly mobile, making them ideally suited for dispersal and reproduction. The growth rate of both larval and adult amphibians is highly variable among species, and in many, it is timed to coincide with favorable environmental conditions.[10] It is thought that for most amphibians growth continues throughout life but slows considerably once they reach adulthood.[14] Similar patterns in growth can be expected to be observed in captive specimens in response to husbandry.

The major morphologic change associated with senescence in amphibians is the accumulation of age pigments. In particular, melanin is produced in regions of high metabolism and is frequently observed in large amounts in the liver. Similarly, granules of sudanophilic lipofuscin can be identified in the neurons of aged toads.[14] Interestingly, the number of nephrons also increase with age, in response to continued body enlargement.[14] Physiologically, increased age is associated with a decrease in metabolic rate, an increase in the cross-linkages of collagen with a subsequent decrease in organ function, and a decrease in the regenerative capacity of amphibians.[14]

Given the variability in growth rates of amphibians in response to external factors, accurately determining the age of unknown individuals is almost impossible in the live animal. However, in deceased amphibians, counting layers in the calcified tissues can be used for age estimations. Most commonly, the bones preferred for this technique include the parasphenoid,[15] zygapophyse of vertebrae,[16] and the pterygoid.[17] In live animals, the bones of phalanges have also been used for age estimation from toe-clipped amphibians,[18] but it is this author's personal opinion that this method is unethical. Annual growth layers in the bones of amphibians appear as wide bands of calcified tissue bordered by resting lines and are a reflection of the seasonal changes in the growth rate of an animal.[18] Longevity of individuals and populations/generations of amphibians is also highly variable and heavily influenced by climactic factors.[18] In general, relatively long lifespans are reported for larger species, whereas small-sized amphibians are short-lived.[14] **Table 1** provides some data on longevity of wild amphibian species.

REPRODUCTION, GROWTH, AND AGING IN REPTILES

Reptile reproductive strategies are varied and range from oviparity to complete viviparity, with the birth of relatively well-developed neonates. The evolutionary transition from egg-laying to live birth has multiple independent origins in squamates but has never developed in any of the other reptile groups.[19] For most reptiles, offspring are precocious and generally are left to fend for themselves, with little to no parental care. Similar to amphibians, growth rate in reptiles is indeterminate and heavily influenced by external factors such as availability of food and water and environmental conditions.[20] Generally speaking, differences exist in growth rates between reptilian orders, but for all reptiles, weight-specific growth rates are lower than those of mammals or birds of comparable size.[20] In addition, there is also variability in the time to reach maturity between reptile orders, with squamates reaching maturity earliest, followed by crocodilians, and then chelonians, with sea turtles taking the longest of any species.[21]

Reptiles seem to show 3 types of senescence; rapid aging and death at mating, gradual senescence comparable to that seen in most of the vertebrates (most squamates), and continued growth throughout life with negligible senescence (chelonians and crocodilians).[22] Changes associated with senility in reptiles may include a decrease in reproductive output (not consistent across all species), a decline in growth rate, accumulation of age pigments, in particular lipofuscin in spinal ganglions and melanism, a decline in metabolic rate, involution of organs and pathology associated with decreased organ function, and a decline in self-regenerative abilities.[22] Physiologically there may be changes in hematology and biochemistry values, tissue and mitochondrial respiration, an increase in calcification, particularly of the growth plates in long bones, and an increase in the number of cross-linkages of collagen proteins.[22]

Table 1
Longevity of selected wild amphibians

Species	Maximal Age (y)
Fischer's clawed salamander (*Onychodactylus fischeri*)	17
Siberian salamander (*Salamandrella keyserlingii*)	8
Eastern newt (*Notophthalmus viridescens*)	9
Pyrenean brook salamander (*Euproctus asper*)	20–26
Alpine salamander (*Salamandra atra*)	15–17
Alpine newt (*Triturus alpestris*)	9–10
Smooth newt (*Triturus vulgaris*)	12
Northern crested newt (*Triturus cristatus*)	14–16
Marbled newt (*Triturus marmoratus*)	14–16
Bosca's newt (*Triturus boscai*)	8
Italian crested newt (*Triturus carnifex*)	9–11
Himalayan newt (*Tylototriton verrucosus*)	11
Tailed frog (*Ascaphus truei*)	14
Oriental fire-bellied toad (*Bombina orientalis*)	12–13
European fire-bellied toad (*Bombina bombina*)	11
Common toad (*Bufo bufo*)	9–12
American toad (*Bufo americanus*)	5
Argentine common toad (*Bufo arenarum*)	8
Penton's toad (*Bufo pentoni*)	6
Spring peeper (*Pseudacris crucifer*)	4
Common frog (*Rana temporaria*)	11–14
Moor frog (*Rana arvalis*)	10–12
Marsh frog (*Rana ridibunda*)	10–12
Pool frog (*Rana lessonae*)	6
Edible frog (*Rana esculenta*)	12
Siberian wood frog (*Rana amurensis*)	9
Long-legged wood frog (*Rana macrocnemis*)	5
Iberian frog (*Rana iberica*)	8
Perez's frog (*Rana perezi*)	5
Northern leopard frog (*Rana pipiens*)	5

Adapted from Smirina EM. Age determination and longevity in amphibians. Gerontology 1994;40:133-46.

Longevity of reptiles varies considerably between species; however, it should be noted that within this taxon are some of the most long-lived animals on the plant. There are reports of some species of chelonians surviving for more than 150 years,[23] and it is important that clients be made aware of this before purchasing a reptile, as there is the potential for a substantial investment in time for the length of the animal's life. Clients who are not prepared for this should be dissuaded from keeping particularly long-lived species such as chelonians. Similar to amphibians, determining age in reptiles with an unknown history is almost impossible in the living animal, but sclerochronology and counting of annular growth rings in the boney tissues have been well described for a range of reptiles.[23] Longevity of reptiles is influenced by a range of external factors, but roughly speaking the Amphisbaenia are the shortest lived, followed in order by

Serpentes, Lacertilia, Crocodilia, Sphenodontidae, and Chelonia.[23] **Table 2** provides some data on longevity of wild reptilian species.

CLINICAL CONSIDERATIONS FOR GERIATRIC AMPHIBIANS AND REPTILES

Geriatric medicine is a poorly described discipline in reptile and amphibian medicine, with few disease processes linked exclusively to senescence. As with most of the

Table 2 Longevity of selected wild reptiles	
Species	Ecological Age (y)
Leopard fringe-fingered lizard (Acanthodactylus pardalis)	3–4
Simon's desert racer (Mesalina olivieri)	5
Atlantic lizard (Gallotia atlantica)	5–6
Gallot's lizard (Gallotia galloti)	7–8
Gran Canaria giant lizard (Gallotia stehlini)	11–12
Sand lizard (Lacerta agilis)	4–5
Ocellated lizard (Lacerta lepida)	10
European green lizard (Lacerta viridis)	6
Viviparous lizard (Lacerta vivipara)	3–4
Iberian wall lizard (Podarcis hispanica)	3
Common wall lizard (Podarcis muralis)	9–11
Rusty-rumped whiptail (Cnemidophorus scalaris)	3
Oriental garden lizard (Calotes versicolor)	4
Peninsular rock agama (Psammophilus dorsalis)	3–4
Greater earless lizard (Cophosaurus texanus)	3–4
Green iguana (Iguana iguana)	9
Desert monitor (Varanus griseus)	8–10
Nile monitor (Varanus niloticus)	8–9
Moorish gecko (Tarentola mauritanica)	8–9
Tuatara (Sphenodon punctatus)	30–35
Ladder snake (Elaphe scalaris)	15–16
Montpellier snake (Malpolon monspessulanus)	18–20
Grass snake (Natrix natrix)	16–19
Habu snake (Trimeresurus flavoviridis)	7–14
Okinawa pitviper (Trimeresurus okinawensis)	15–19
European asp (Vipera aspis)	15–18
Greek tortoise (Testudo graeca)	19–20
Hermann's tortoise (Testudo hermanni)	18–20
Painted turtle (Chrysemys picta)	20
European pond turtle (Emys orbicularis)	16
Common snapping turtle (Chelydra serpentina)	20
Loggerhead turtle (Caretta caretta)	75–80
Nile crocodile (Crocodylus niloticus)	40–50
Siamese crocodile (Crocodylus siamensis)	12
Alligator (Alligator mississippiensis)	22–25

Adapted from Castanet J. Age estimation and longevity in reptiles. Gerontology 1994;40:174-92.

illnesses seen in these species, husbandry plays a large role both in their onset and in determining successful recovery. Inappropriate husbandry may be the primary cause, or it may be that animals are being provided adequate husbandry, but due to other disease processes they are unable to use their environment properly, leading to secondary husbandry deficiencies. A key component of any herptile veterinary examination, regardless of the animals age, is obtaining a thorough history and signalment, which may give the clinician an indication of the principal cause for the presenting complaint. Regular examination, including serial diagnostics (radiographs, hematology, and biochemistry), of individual animals may be invaluable in categorizing decline, as there is a lack of normal data for many herptiles, and there can be great difficulty in interpreting one-off results because of the fluctuating nature of blood parameters in these species due to a range of uncontrollable variables such as season, diet, sex, environment, and reproductive status.[24–27] This can allow the clinician to tailor their approach to the individual needs of their patients and may provide an early warning system for detecting abnormalities in organ function and aid in revealing the presence of degenerative diseases such as osteoarthritis, spondylopathy, dystrophic and metastatic mineralization, uroliths, organomegaly, neoplasia, cataracts, and other masses. Irrespective of the disease process, successful management of elderly patients requires a combination of medical or surgical intervention, coupled with appropriate changes to husbandry, which may include modifications to enclosures that take into consideration the physical abilities of geriatric individuals. With advancements in the efficacy and safety of both injectable and inhalant anaesthetics for reptiles and amphibians, clinicians should not be fearful of sedating senescent animals in order to facilitate diagnosis and treatment. **Table 3** briefly summarizes some of the most common ailments that afflict geriatric herpetofauna; however, it should be noted that this list is by no means exhaustive.

ASSESSMENT OF QUALITY OF LIFE

Assessment of quality of life in reptiles and amphibians may be difficult, as they are typically stoic in nature and adept at masking illness. Furthermore, the highly subjective nature of animal assessments, coupled with other extraneous factors such as perceived worth (genetics, appearance, monetary), means that there is the risk of profound suffering and poor animal welfare outcomes in these groups, particularly under circumstances where animals are not regularly examined or kept by inexperienced hobbyists. In order to circumvent this, it is recommended that clinicians establish an objective set of criteria against which they wish to rank the quality of an individual's life. The Association of Zoos and Aquariums (www.aza.org) recommends the use of median life expectancy as the primary referenced statistical for species longevity, and they provide data on the life expectancy of a small number of herpetofauna. Another useful resource for clinicians is the website Animal Diversity Web (www.animaldiversity.org),[38] which has greater detail on life history traits, including life expectancy, for a wide range of animals. When no captive life expectancy data are available, closely related species, or the wild lifespan, can be used as a guide with the understanding that for most species, the captive lifespan should be significantly longer than wild lifespan.

A comprehensive quality-of-life assessment should take into consideration factors such as behavior, social standing, and existing medical conditions. Once completed for an individual, the assessment needs to be stored, and reviewed at regular intervals, or reassessed if there has been a noticeable change or decline in the animal's demeanor. An example of a quality-of-life assessment document has been provided in **Table 4**. Possible outcomes of a quality-of-life assessment may include euthanasia,

Table 3
Summary of medical conditions seen in senescent amphibians and reptiles

Organ System	Disease	Clinical Signs and Diagnosis	Treatment
Integument	Dysecdysis (Fig. 1)	Presence of retained sections of skin, missing digits or tail tips, retained spectacles (snakes and geckoes).	Remove retained portions of skin. Improve husbandry (increase humidity, provide structures for rubbing). Hematology and biochemistry to check if secondary to organ dysfunction.
Gastrointestinal	Overgrown rhamphothecae	Typically presents as an overbite or distortion of the beak.	Debridement of overgrown portions, correct underlying husbandry.
	Periodontal disease (Fig. 2)	Most commonly seen in acrodont species (Agamidae and Chamaeleonidae).[28] Gingivitis, loss of teeth, osteomyelitis of the jaw bones.	Debridement of lesions including dental scale and administration of both topical and systemic antimicrobials. Correct deficiencies in diet.[28]
	Constipation	Physical examination and history, radiographs. May be primary GIT disease or secondary to renomegaly or physical deformation (eg, narrowing of pelvic canal).	Correct underlying husbandry deficits (diet, hydration, supplements). Supportive therapy including fluids, provision of heat and warm soaks, enema in severe cases. Investigate causes of renomegaly and morphologic deformations.
Musculoskeletal	Osteoarthritis	Joint swelling, loss of range of movement, reluctance to move. Diagnosis with radiographs/CT.	Provision of analgesia, in severe cases involving a single limb, amputation may be warranted. Modification of enclosure so animal still able to reach basking areas etc.
	Spondylopathy	Most frequently seen in snakes, especially sedentary, obese individuals. Manifested as a reluctance to move or stiffness when slithering and climbing. Diagnosis with radiographs/CT.	Provision of analgesia, weight loss, modification of enclosure.

(continued on next page)

Table 3
(continued)

Organ System	Disease	Clinical Signs and Diagnosis	Treatment
	Articular gout	Joint swelling, reluctance to move. Typically, a sequalae to renal failure in reptiles. Diagnosis with radiographs/CT, aspirates of affected joints, and renal biopsy. Biochemistry is rarely of value, as uric acid levels are not necessarily an accurate measure of renal function in reptiles.[29]	Fluid therapy and diuresis, xanthine oxidase inhibitors, dietary adjustments, analgesia.[30]
	Renal secondary hyperparathyroidism	Physical deformity, pain or reluctance to move, pathologic fractures. Diagnosis with radiographs/CT, hematology and biochemistry, renal biopsy.	Provision of analgesia, stabilization of fractures, treatment of renal disease.
	Muscle atrophy	Common in sedentary individuals. May be a precursor to secondary ailments such as spondylopathy and reproductive disorders.	Modify enclosure design to encourage movement, regularly remove animals from enclosures for physiotherapy sessions such as swimming or free climbing.
Cardiovascular	Atherosclerosis and dystrophic myocardial mineralization	Failure to thrive, neuropathies if blood vessels of the CNS are involved, peracute death. Diagnosis best made with ultrasound.	The efficacy of cholesterol-lowering drugs in these species is unknown.[31]
Urinary	Renal disease (**Fig. 3**)	May manifest as articular or visceral gout and clinical signs depend on site of crystal deposition.	Fluid therapy and diuresis, xanthine oxidase inhibitors (eg, allopurinol), dietary adjustments, analgesia.
	Urolithiasis (**Fig. 4**)	Dysuria, stranguria, hematuria, lethargy, and inappetence. Diagnosis with radiographs. Be aware that in some species (particularly chelonians) retropulsion of retained eggs into the bladder is a common sequalae to administration of oxytocin to dystocic animals.[32]	Removal of the foreign body via endoscopy or traditional surgical approaches.

Reproductive	Follicular stasis, dystocia, and egg coelomitis (Fig. 5)	History of observed nesting without production of eggs or offspring, lethargy, and general malaise. Diagnosis with hematology and biochemistry, cytology, and imaging such as radiographs, ultrasound, and CT.	A combination of medical management and surgical intervention depending on the severity and nature of disease.
	Infection or impaction of hemipenal pockets	Swelling of the tail base.	Removal of plugs or debridement of abscessed material and administration of antimicrobials as necessary.
Neurologic	Cerebral xanthomatosis	Incoordination, ataxia, opisthotonos, loss of righting reflex, tremors, and seizures.	Have been reported in a range of squamates with no known successful case outcomes.[33–35]
Endocrine	Nutritional secondary hypothyroidism	Presumptive cases have been seen in herbivorous lizards and chelonians in response to low dietary iodine.[36] Clinical signs may include edema of the neck, head, and forelimbs as well as general malaise. Definitive diagnosis is difficult as serum T4 levels are poorly described in reptiles.	Correct underlying dietary deficiencies, supplementation with iodine not usually necessary and may result in goiter.[36]
Special senses	Lipid keratopathy, cataracts (Fig. 6)	Lipid deposits in the cornea of a variety of species have been reported including amphibians and squamate reptiles. Poorly defined pathophysiology with several risk factors identified, including obesity and higher incidence in female animals. Cataracts may be present as clouding/complete opacity of the lens leading to blindness.	Treatment is rarely rewarding, and animals have marked reduction in visual acuity leading to eventual blindness. Snakes with cataracts may be presented deceased prey with tweezers and many will eat when this technique is used.
All body systems	Neoplasia (Figs. 7 and 8)	A wide array of neoplastic conditions has been reported in all body systems for both amphibians and reptiles, and clinical signs may depend on the type of neoplasm and organ affected.	Treatment options include surgery, chemotherapy, and radiation therapy.[37]

Data from references in the table.

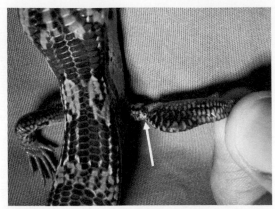

Fig. 1. Dysecdysis can cause annular constrictions on limbs and in severe cases can lead to limb amputation, such as in this pink-tongued skink (*Cyclodomorphus gerrardii*).

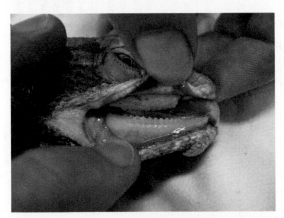

Fig. 2. Severe cases of periodontal disease may lead to loss of sections of the dental arcade, such as the missing portion of the maxilla in this central bearded dragon (*Pogona vitticeps*).

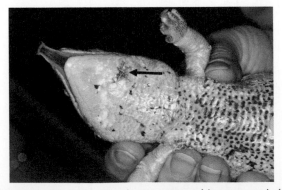

Fig. 3. Dermal metastatic mineralization in an eastern blue-tongued skink (Tiliqua scincoides) secondary to chronic renal failure. (*Arrow* points to biopsy site).

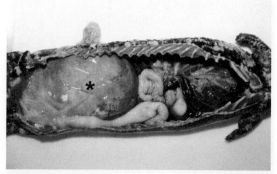

Fig. 4. Large urolith in the bladder of a shingleback lizard (*Tiliqua rugosa*). (Cranial is to the right). *, Urolith.

continued monitoring with the use of a quality-of-life plan, or more detailed veterinary investigation.

EUTHANASIA

For all living beings, death is a natural conclusion to life, and a vital aspect of the veterinary profession is the provision of euthanasia. The euthanasia of animals carries

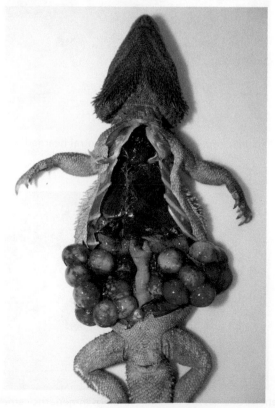

Fig. 5. Follicular stasis in a central bearded dragon.

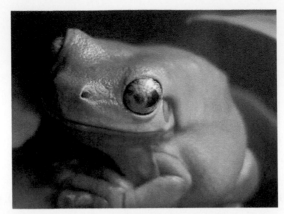

Fig. 6. Lipid keratopathy in a green tree frog (*Litoria caerulea*).

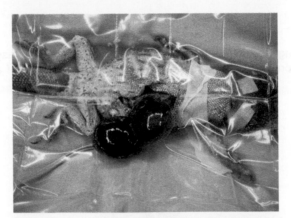

Fig. 7. Undescribed hepatic neoplasm in a geriatric central bearded dragon.

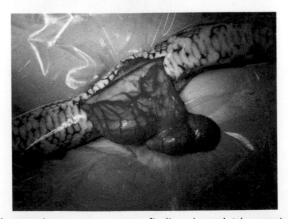

Fig. 8. Gastric adenocarcinomas are common findings in geriatric carpet pythons (*Morelia spilota*).

Table 4
Example of a quality-of-life assessment document

Quality of Life Assessment			

Date:_____   Life Expectancy:_____
Species:_____
Current Age:_____

Behavioral Parameters		Weighting	Score
Lame or stiff gait	1 = Mild. 5 = Severe.	x 2	
Lethargy or reduced mental alertness	1 = Mild. 5 = Severe.	x 2	
Mobility (ability to stand on hind legs, jump, climb, move in coordinated way)	1 = Mild reduction. 5 = Marked reduction	x 2	
Activity (willingness to forage or explore enclosure)	1 = Mild reduction. 5 = Marked reduction	x 2	
Motivation (willingness to take part in rewarding activities)	1 = Mild reduction. 5 = Marked reduction		
Appetite	1 = Mild reduction. 5 = Marked reduction	x 2	
Urinary or fecal incontinence	Always score 5 if incontinence is seen	x 2	
Behaviors resulting in self-trauma (eg, repetitive scratching, licking, biting)	3 = Mild. 5 = Severe	x 2	
Apparent loss of vision	1 = Presumed mild reduction (eg, senile nuclear sclerosis). 5 = Appears blind.		
Weakness (lack of muscle strength)	1 = Mild. 5 = Severe.		
Any other unusual behavior	Specify behavior and score 1–5.		
TOTAL for behavioral parameters			

Social Parameters - Disregard if Solitary Species		Weighting	Score
Target for aggression	0 = No. 2 = Mild/infrequent aggression. 5 = Severe/ frequent aggression.	x 2	
Ostracized from group	0 = No. 3 = Yes.	x 2	
Perceived to have a positive role in social structure	0 = Yes (or not applicable). 1 = No.		

(*continued on next page*)

Table 4 (continued)			
Social Parameters - Disregard if Solitary Species		**Weighting**	**Score**
Shows inappropriate social behaviors meaning has to be permanently isolated from group	No = 0. Yes, but does not seem to affect quality of life = 1. Yes and does seem to affect quality of life = 5.		
Animal is a social species but can only be housed alone due to no available conspecifics	No = 0. Yes = 5		
Animal is a social species, is aged, and is kept isolated but would have to move to another zoo in order to be in a social group	No move required or no concern about how animal would cope with move = 0. Yes, move needed, and there is concern that move would affect quality of life = 5		
TOTAL for social parameters			
Medical Parameters		**Weighting**	**Score**
Body condition score or weight	0 = ideal, 5 = poor (either emaciated or obese)	x 2	
Osteoarthritis:			
Single joint	3 = mild, 5 = severe	x 2	
Multiple joint	3 = mild, 5 = severe	x 2	
Spondylosis or other spinal disease	3 = mild, 5 = severe	x 2	
Anemia or white blood cell abnormality	3 = mild, 5 = severe	x 2	
Kidney disease	3 = mild, 5 = severe	x 2	
Cardiovascular disease	3 = mild, 5 = severe	x 2	
Respiratory disease	3 = mild, 5 = severe	x 2	
Liver disease	3 = mild, 5 = severe	x 2	
Malignancy	3 = mild, 5 = severe	x 2	
Ongoing neurologic signs	3 = mild, 5 = severe	x 2	
Diabetes	Always score 5	x 2	
Animal has a zoonotic or communicable disease	No = 0, Yes = 5	x 2	
Dental disease (worn or missing teeth, periodontal disease)	0 = normal dentition, 1 = mild disease or one tooth missing, 5 = severe disease or more than half of the teeth missing		
Reproductive disease	3 = mild, 5 = severe		

(continued on next page)

Table 4
(continued)

Medical Parameters		Weighting	Score
Ocular disease	3 = mild (eg, slightly reduced vision, intermittent keratitis), 5 = severe (eg: presumed blind, chronic keratitis)		
Skin disease	1 = mild, 5 = severe		
Animal has disease that requires medications	No = 0. Daily or occasional medication required without animal restraint = 0. Occasional (multiple times per year) medication requiring manual restraint/ darting = 1. Daily medication requiring restraint for short treatment course (<7 d) = 2. Daily medication requiring restraint for longer period (>7 d) = 3–4. Daily medication requiring restraint every day for the rest of the animal's life = 5.		
Animal has disease that requires invasive surgery	3 = Invasive surgery with good prognosis. 4 = Invasive surgery with fair prognosis. 5 = Invasive surgery with guarded to poor prognosis.		
Other significant disease process	Specify disease and score severity from 1–5		
TOTAL for medical parameters			
RESULTS			
Total Quality of Life Score today _____	Guide to interpreting results SOCIAL SPECIES Acceptable welfare: score 0–35 Questionable welfare: score 35–50 Unacceptable welfare: score >50 SOLITARY SPECIES Acceptable welfare: score 0–30 Questionable welfare: score 30–45 Unacceptable welfare: score >45		
Compare with previous scores	Date Date Date		

Adapted from Zoos Victoria, Courtesy of S. Frith, BVSc MVS, Melbourne, Australia.

significant professional, moral, and ethical responsibilities for veterinarians. All animals deserve a dignified death, free of fear and pain, conducted in a humane manner in accordance with local laws. With this in mind, each veterinarian has to determine the process for euthanasia that sits most comfortably with them and takes into consideration the anatomic and physiologic diversity of the herpetofauna. No matter the species or circumstances, it is typically this author's preference to sedate all animals before euthanasia. Administration of either tiletamine/zolazepam, 50 mg/kg, intramuscularly (IM) or subcutaneously (SQ), or ketamine HCL, 100 mg/kg, IM or SQ, will generally result in deep sedation in most of the herptile species. Once the sedation has taken effect, intravenous, intracardiac, or intracranial administration of euthanasia solution (most commonly pentobarbital sodium) can be administered.[39] Alternatively, once the animal is anesthetized, a physical method of euthanasia can be applied, such as penetrating captive bolt, blunt force trauma to the head, firearm, or pithing. Hypothermia is not considered a humane method of euthanasia for any amphibian or reptile species.[39] For a more comprehensive review of euthanasia techniques of herpetofauna refer to the section on end-of-life decisions and euthanasia for exotic animals in this edition. No matter the method of euthanasia, it is worth mentioning that in reptiles and amphibians, there may be significant lag time from death of the animal to asystole, such that in some cases the heart may continue to beat for hours following clinical death of the patient. Owners should be made aware of this before euthanasia to avoid any confusion, as it may be possible for them to visualize a beating heart despite the animal being pronounced dead.

SUMMARY

Reptiles and amphibians have steadily captured the imagination of pet owners the world over. For many hobbyists, they are now considered mainstream pets and are valued and integral components of the family unit. As a profession, veterinarians have to be acutely aware of the strong bonds formed between captive herpetofauna and their owners and work closely with them to devise life-long health plans, especially in species with extended life expectancies. As reptiles and amphibians age, their welfare requires careful, ongoing assessment, and adjustments may need to be made to their husbandry and medical management in order to accommodate any frailties associated with senescence. Most importantly, under circumstances where an elderly amphibian or reptile is approaching the end of its life, its death needs to be facilitated with the compassion and humanness that should be afforded to all species.

DISCLOSURE

The author has nothing to disclose.

REFERENCES

1. Schoch RR. Amphibian evolution: the life of early land vertebrates. West Sussex (United Kingdom): Wiley Blackwell; 2014.
2. Laurin M, Reisz RR. A reevaluation of early amniote phylogeny. Zoo J Linn Soc 1995;113:165–223.
3. Wake DB, Koo MS. Amphibians. Curr Biol 2018;28:R1237–41.
4. Uetz P, Freed P, Hošek J. The reptile database. 2018. Available at: www.reptile-database.org. Accessed January 09, 2019.
5. Böhm M, Collen B, Baillie JEM, et al. The conservation status of the world's reptiles. Biol Cons 2013;157:372–85.
6. AVMA. U.S. pet ownership statistics. 2019. Available at: https://www.avma.org/KB/Resources/Statistics/Pages/Market-research-statistics-US-pet-ownership.aspx. Accessed January 09, 2019.
7. Zhang P, Zhou H, Chen YQ, et al. Mitogenomic perspectives on the origin and phylogeny of living amphibians. Syst Biol 2005;54:391–400.

8. Modesto SP, Anderson JS. The phylogenetic definition of reptilia. Syst Biol 2004; 53:815–21.
9. Pincheira-Donoso1 D, Bauer AM, Meiri S, et al. Global taxonomic diversity of living reptiles. PLOS One 2013;8:e59741.
10. Hota AK. Growth in amphibians. Gerontology 1994;40:147–60.
11. Rowlands IW, Weir BJ. The ovarian cycle in vertebrates. In: Zuckerman L, Barbara JW, editors. The ovary. 22nd edition. New York: Academic Press; 1977. p. 217–73.
12. Amoroso EC. Placentation. In: Parkes AS, editor. Marshall's physiology of reproduction. London: Longmans Green; 1952. p. 127–311.
13. Lamotte M, Rey P, Vogeli M. Reseches sur l'ovaire de *Nectophrynoides orientalis*, Batracien anoure vivipare. Arch Anat Microsc Morphol Exp 1964;53:179–234.
14. Kara TC. Ageing in amphibians. Gerontology 1994;40:161–73.
15. Senning WC. A study of age determination and growth of *Necturus maculosus* based on the parasphenoid bone. Am J Anat 1940;66:483–94.
16. Willis YL. Breeding transformation and determination of age of the bullfrog (*Rana catesbeiana* Shaw) in Missouri. Columbia: University of Missouri; 1954.
17. Schroeder EE, Baskett T. Age estimation, growth rates and population structure in Missouri bullfrogs. Copeia 1968;3:583–92.
18. Smirina EM. Age determination and longevity in amphibians. Gerontology 1994; 40:133–46.
19. Rafferty A, Evans R, Scheelings T, et al. Limited oxygen availability in utero may constrain the evolution of live birth in reptiles. Am Nat 2013;181:245–53.
20. Avery RA. Growth in reptiles. Gerontology 1994;40:193–9.
21. Scott R, Marsh R, Hays GC. Life in the really slow lane: loggerhead sea turtles mature late relative to other reptiles. Funct Ecol 2012;26:227–35.
22. Patnaik BK. Ageing in Reptiles. Gerontology 1994;40:200–20.
23. Castanet J. Age estimation and longevity in reptiles. Gerontology 1994;40: 174–92.
24. Campbell TW, Ellis CK. Hematology of reptiles. In: Campbell TW, Ellis CK, editors. Avian and exotic animal hematology and cytology. 3rd edition. Ames (IA): Blackwell Publishing; 2007. p. 3–82.
25. Scheelings TF, Rafferty AR. Hematologic and serum biochemical values of gravid freshwater Australian chelonians. J Wildl Dis 2012;48:314–21.
26. Scheelings TF, Williamson SA, Reina RD. Hematology and serum biochemistry for free-ranging freshwater crocodiles (*Crocodylus johnstoni*) in Western Australia. J Wildl Dis 2016;52:959–61.
27. Scheelings T, Jessop T. Influence of capture method, habitat quality and individual traits on blood parameters of free-ranging lace monitors (*Varanus varius*). Aust Vet J 2011;89:360–5.
28. McCracken H, Birch CA. Periodontal disease in lizards. In: Murray REM, Fowler E, editors. Zoo and wildlife animal medicine. Philadelphia: WB Saunders Co; 1999. p. 252–7.
29. Hernandez-Divers SJ. Endoscopic renal evaluation and biopsy of chelonia. Vet Rec 2004;154:73–80.
30. Divers SJ, Innis CJ. Urology. In: Divers SJ, Stahl SJ, editors. Mader's reptile and amphibian medicine and surgery. 3rd edition. St Louis (MO): Elsevier; 2019. p. 626–48.
31. Paré JA, Lentini AM. Reptile geriatrics. Vet Clin North Am Exot Anim Pract 2010; 13:15–25.

32. Minter LJ, Wood MW, Hill TL, et al. Cystoscopic guided removal of ectopic eggs from the urinary bladder of the Florida cooter turtle (*Pseudemys floridana floridana*). J Zoo Widl Med 2010;41:503–9.
33. Anderson ET, Troan BV, Stringer EM, et al. Cerebral xanthoma in a long-nosed snake (*Rhinocheilus lecontei*). J Herpetol Med Surg 2010;20:58–60.
34. Garner MM, Lung NP, Murray S. Xanthomatosis in geckos: five cases. J Zoo Widl Med 1999;30:443–7.
35. Kummrow MS, Berkvens CN, Paré JA, et al. Cerebral xanthomatosis in three green water dragons (*Physignathus cocincinus*). J Zoo Widl Med 2010;41: 128–32.
36. Mans C, Braun J. Update on common nutritional disorders of captive reptiles. Vet Clin North Am Exot Anim Pract 2014;17:369–95.
37. Christman J, Devau M, Wilson-Robles H, et al. Oncology of reptiles: diseases, diagnosis, and treatment. Vet Clin North Am Exot Anim Pract 2017;20:87–110.
38. Myers P, Espinosa R, Parr CS, et al. Animal Diversity Web. 2019. Available at: http://www.animaldiversity.org. Accessed January 09, 2019.
39. Nevarez JG. Euthanasia. In: Divers SJ, Stahl SJ, editors. Mader's reptile and amphibian medicine and surgery. 3rd edition. St Louis (MO): Elsevier; 2019. p. 437–40.

Care of the Geriatric Raptor

John Chitty, BVetMed, CertZooMed, MRCVS

KEYWORDS

- Raptor • Geriatric • Welfare • Captive • Owl

KEY POINTS

- Older or geriatric raptors are frequently housed in zoologic collections or maintained by falconers.
- Diseases such as osteoarthritis and those affecting the special senses are common and may impact welfare without overt clinical signs.
- Careful management and husbandry of these older birds can produce a positive welfare benefit for them.
- Regular monitoring and quality-of-life assessments are important to recognize and manage potentially painful conditions.

WHAT IS A RAPTOR?

A raptor is generally defined as carnivorous birds that are members of the Falconiformes.[1] This includes:

- Cathartidae—New World Vultures
- Pandionidae—the Osprey
- Acciptridae—hawks, eagles and Old World Vultures
- Sagittaridae—the Secretary Bird
- Falconidae—falcons and caracaras

This definition does not include owls, because these are birds unrelated although they share such characteristics as being carnivores and catching prey with their feet. For the purposes of clarity, and because geriatric owls are frequently found in collections alongside raptors suffering similar problems, members of the Strigiformes[2] (Tytonidae [Barn owls] and Strigidae ["true" owls]) will be included in this article, and the term "raptor" will be used to include owls as well as "true" raptors.

REASONS FOR KEEPING

Raptors have been kept and trained for hunting for thousands of years by many different cultures across the world.[3–5] Falconry is now included on the UNESCO

Anton Vets, Anton Mill Road, Andover, Hants SP10 2NJ, UK
E-mail address: exotics@antonvets.co.uk

Vet Clin Exot Anim 23 (2020) 503–523
https://doi.org/10.1016/j.cvex.2020.05.003
1094-9194/20/© 2020 Elsevier Inc. All rights reserved.

Intangible Cultural Heritage List.[6] Although much of this hunting has been for "the pot" gathering food to feed the falconer and family, at the upper echelons of society, falconry has been principally a sport. As such, it has generated much published material on the keeping of birds and the art of training and flying them.[3–5,7] In more recent times, with the decreasing numbers of raptor species in the wild, there has been much more emphasis on captive breeding and rearing of these species.[3]

A neglected subject in the vast majority of these books is the fate of the older bird with an exception being Cooper (2002).[5] Speaking with falconers there have, traditionally, been various outcomes for older birds in falconry.

- They do not get old. Salvin and Brodrick (1855)[8] state peregrines living to 5 to 8 years old. We are aware peregrines (*Falco peregrinus*) can live much longer than this (discussed elsewhere in this article), and it can be taken as an improvement in husbandry and welfare standards that birds of this age would now be considered young mature birds.
- They are not retained in captivity till old age. Cultures that use "passage" birds for falconry will take chicks from the nest, train them, and then release them after they have been hunted.[9]
- They do not retire. Many falconers do not retire their birds. Although their birds may be flown less or at smaller easier quarry as they get older, their essential husbandry remains the same. The changes in how they are flown, however, suggest recognition of age-related disease or an increased rate of injury. However, such birds are not presented more frequently to the veterinarian for routine health screening, as may be expected.
- They are retired into aviaries. This step is usually for breeding purposes, but may also simply be seclusion flights. In these cases, a lack of environmental enrichment may be an issue, as may be reduced observation and handling.

In recognition of their conservation status, raptors are also frequently kept in zoologic collections. These birds may be kept as falconry birds and used for demonstration purposes, but many are kept in breeding aviaries their entire lives. With minimal threat, these birds may attain older ages (discussed elsewhere in this article), although a lack of handling and observation may decrease the recognition of geriatric disease and so represent a negative welfare situation.

LONGEVITY IN THE WILD AND CAPTIVITY

For species that have been maintained in captivity for so long, and are extensively studied in the wild, data on longevity are not extensive. **Table 1** provides a summary of recorded ages in the wild and in captivity of various species. This list is by no means complete, but includes representative species and sizes of birds. The data from the wild are most contemporary, representing material from regularly updated ornithological societies. Nonetheless, much of these data come from recovered banded birds, many of whom have not died from age-related disease. However, captive data are extremely sparse and the references found are dated. Within the falconry industry, much of the longevity data are anecdotal and this may explain some of the extreme figures quoted by Heidenreich (1997).[10] It is therefore likely that zoo data are more accurate. Interestingly, there seems to be little difference in longevity between sexes, and female birds are often recorded as laying into older age. It is surprising that, where there are reasonable data, there seems to be little difference in longevity records between captive and wild birds, when it might be expected for the former to be longer lived. However, this may be due to the data presented representing extreme ages

Table 1
Longevity of various raptor species

Species	Longevity, Wild (Europe)	Longevity, Wild (UK)	Longevity, Wild (N America)	Captivity
Turkey vulture *Cathartes aura*	—	—	16 y 10 m	21 y
American black vulture *Coargyps atratus*	—	—	25 y	21 y
Black-shouldered kite *Elanus caerulus*	—	—	—	12 y
Brahminy kite *Haliastur indus*	—	—	—	21 y
Red kite *Milvus milvus*	25 y 8 m	25 y 8 m	—	38 y
African fish eagle *Haliaeetus vocifer*	—	—	—	21 y
White-tailed sea eagle *Haliaeetus albicilla*	29 y 10 m	16 y 9 m	—	95 y
Bald eagle *Haliaeetus leucocephalus*	—	—	38 y	36 y
Oriental white-backed vulture *Gyps bengalensis*	—	—	—	23 y
Griffon vulture *Gyps fulvus*	9 y 11 m	—	—	31 y
European black vulture *Aegypius monachus*	—	—	—	26 y
Northern goshawk *Accipiter gentilis*	22 y	18 y 8 m	16 y 10 m	24 y >28 y
Red-tailed hawk *Buteo jamaicensis*	—	—	30y 8 m	23 y
Common buzzard *Buteo buteo*	28 y 9 m	30y 5 m	—	15 y
Harris' hawk *Parabuteo unicinctus*	—	—	15 y	25 y
Tawny eagle *Aquila rapax*	—	—	—	23 y
Golden eagle *Aquila chrysaetos*	>32 y	16 y	31 y 8 m	>48 y
Secretary bird *Sagittarius serpentarius*	—	—	—	18 y
Saker falcon *Falco cherrug*	15 y 11 m	—	—	29 y
Peregrine falcon *Falco peregrinus*	17 y 4 m	21 y 10 m	19 y 9 m	24 y
Common kestrel *Falco tinnunculus*	20 y 5 m	15 y 11 m	—	14 y
American kestrel *Falco sparverius*			14 y 8 m	

(continued on next page)

Table 1 (continued)				
Species	Longevity, Wild (Europe)	Longevity, Wild (UK)	Longevity, Wild (N America)	Captivity
Barn owl *Tyto alba*	>17 y 11 m	15y 3 m	15 y 5 m	15 y
Great horned owl *Bubo virginianus*	—	—	28 y	22 y
Snowy owl *Bubo scandiacus*	—	—	23 y 10 m	20 y
European eagle owl *Bubo bubo*	27 y 4 m	—	—	5 y

Data from refs.[10–16]

attended rather than mean or median survival age. Cooper[5] (2002) reports zoo-kept birds as living longer than falconry birds.

HOW TO "AGE" A RAPTOR

Much data are based on plumage and concentrates on distinguishing juveniles from subadults from adults. However, there is little ability to distinguish the older, or geriatric, bird. There are a few exceptions, for example, the male Bateleur eagle (*Terathopius ecaudatus*), where paling of the facial skin color may occur in older birds.[16] In Barn owls (*Tyto alba*), talon flanges on digit 3 provide a reasonable estimate of age with the number and depth of notches being used[17] (**Fig. 1**). More recently, pentosidine analysis has been advocated as a means of aging birds and may have applications in forensic and conservation medicine.[18]

AGE AND REASONS FOR RETIREMENT

As stated elsewhere in this article, many birds either do not attain retirement or are not retired. In terms of decision making as to when to retire a falconry bird there is little, if

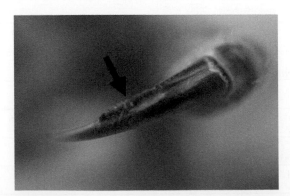

Fig. 1. Talon flanges on a Barn Owl (*Tyto alba*) digit 3. Given the number of flanges and length of flanged talon the bird is more than 2 years old. Wear on the flanges indicates the bird is likely much older than this. Arrow indicates talon flanges.

any, material, with most falconers making an empirical decision based on the bird's flying and hunting abilities, or after an injury. This would suggest that birds are not retired until showing overt signs of age-related disorders, yet this does not seem to be accompanied by an increase in care or veterinary attention, with retired birds generally being placed into aviaries with less handling and observation.

For arthritic birds, although reduced hunting decreases the loading of joints and risk of further injury, a lack of analgesia and likely weight gain (with resultant joint loading) may well result in extended welfare compromise.

As stated elsewhere in this article, some birds are retired into breeding aviaries. However, there is evidence that aging changes may result in reduced fertility.

HUSBANDRY OF THE GERIATRIC BIRD

Other than falconry birds that may be flown, and actively managed, into older age most retired birds or older zoo birds will be housed in aviaries. The management of raptors in aviaries is well-described by Parry-Jones (2008)[19] and is generally minimally invasive with birds rarely handled. Disturbance (cleaning, physical checks, etc) is usually reduced to an as-needed basis.

NUTRITION OF THE RETIRED BIRD

Given the numbers of birds kept worldwide in falconry and the likely number of aged birds flying or retired, it is surprising to find such a paucity of coverage of the older bird in the veterinary literature especially given the amount of description of their ailments and diseases over such a long time.[10,20,21] One of the exceptions is Cooper (2002),[5] where there is a brief outline of potential issues affecting the older bird. A fuller account is given by Tristram (2010).[22]

One aspect highlighted is that of obesity in the older bird.[5] Actively flying birds have dietary intake and body weight/condition tightly monitored.[3,4] This is often not the case in aviary birds, which may suffer a combination of reduced exercise and higher calorie intake. Aviary birds rarely have bodyweight and condition checked as often as flying birds. As such, the older retired bird in an aviary may become obese. This condition may be linked to an increased likelihood of obesity-related conditions, including hepatic lipidosis, atherosclerosis, and bumblefoot[5] (**Figs. 2** and **3**). Increased loading on leg joints may worsen the clinical signs of osteoarthritis. Conversely, appetite is hard to assess in aviary birds with some birds stashing food rather than eating it.

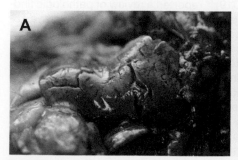
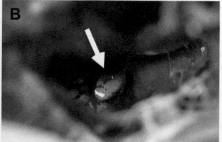

Fig. 2. (*A*) Severe hepatic lipidosis in an owl at post mortem examination. Note the friability of the tissue. (*B*) Fatty changes in the kidney of a Common kestrel (*Falco tinnunculus*) at post mortem examination). Arrow indicates pale kidney.

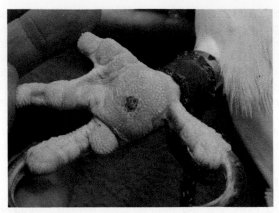

Fig. 3. Bumblefoot (stage 2/3) in a Gyrfalcon (*Falco rusticolus*).

Unless the aviary is regularly and thoroughly inspected, this practice may be hard to detect.

AGE-RELATED DISORDERS

As has been discussed elsewhere in this article, some health conditions may become more likely in the geriatric bird.[23] These conditions are discussed in this section. However, clinicians should always remember that some conditions affect birds of all ages and so should not be forgotten when drawing up differential diagnoses in each case.

When investigating the older bird, there may be other factors to consider, including the likelihood of potential underlying disease to adversely affect recovery from anesthesia.[5] Certainly when planning major surgeries and intervention, a full discussion with the owner should be carried out to establish the likely impact of treatment on the bird; the owner's ability to manage the bird during and after treatment; and a risk-benefit analysis, where the adverse effects of treatment (eg, postsurgical pain, stress of handling for wound management) are weighed against the effects of therapy on the bird's welfare and longevity.

NEOPLASIA

Reports of neoplasia in birds of prey are surprisingly uncommon in the literature given the ages of birds kept in captivity. Chitty (2019)[23] reported a review of pathologic findings from a zoologic collection with only a single (benign) neoplasm found over a 15-year period. In this author's experience, squamous cell carcinoma is the most commonly seen neoplasm in raptors but is normally associated with chronic skin irritation or trauma and is not usually associated with older birds[24] (**Fig. 4**). **Table 2** provides an overview of reported neoplasms in birds of prey.

Therapy of neoplasia is principally surgical excision.[26] Where this is not possible, euthanasia is often advocated. Overall in avian medicine, reports of chemotherapy, photodynamic therapy, or radiation therapy are present, but are usually based on single cases meaning that the results, doses, and technique usually require extrapolation to other species or situations.[22,26] Nonetheless, knowledge of such therapies is increasing in avian medicine and clinicians are recommended to investigate treatment possibilities on a case-by-case basis using the most up-to-date literature.[28,29] Clinicians are also reminded that when using chemotherapies there are considerable

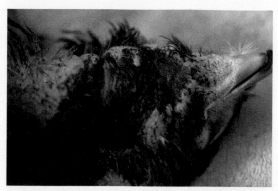

Fig. 4. Squamous cell carcinoma in a Peregrine falcon (*Falco peregrinus*).

health and safety implications to clinic staff and to handlers because it will be uncertain as to how the agent will be excreted nor for how long. Similarly, side effects will be less well-known and potentially more likely when extrapolating dose rates from other nonrelated avian species.[30] As such, full informed owner consent is always required when using these therapies.

OSTEOARTHRITIS

Osteoarthritis is extremely common in older birds, but can be hard to identify or diagnose.[31] As a result, welfare compromise may well occur when painful lesions are not treated or managed. In the author's experience, hips and the intertarsal joints are most commonly affected, with stifles and elbows being next most common. In larger owls, the 2 vertebral joints between the notarium and synsacrum also seem overly represented (**Fig. 5**).

Osteoarthritis is most common, most likely as a result of wear and tear, trauma, or postsepsis damage. However, septic arthritis and, more rarely, articular gout may also be seen.

Clinical signs include:

- Reluctance to fly or walk
- Altered stance or perching
- Bumblefoot (especially unilateral lesion on the opposite limb to the arthritic lesions)
- Weight loss
- Lethargy

On clinical examination, the affected joints may be swollen and hot initially, although this is usually not the case in chronic cases. Joints may be stiff and unable to move through their full range of motion. Birds show evidence of pain on manipulation of affected joints. There may also be muscle wastage around the affected joints, reflecting altered limb use.

Imaging is the primary means of diagnosis, with radiography being the general technique of choice. Soft tissue swelling and joint effusion may be seen in some cases. In more chronic cases, reactive ossification of the surrounding tissues may be seen, as may degenerative changes in the joint surfaces (**Fig. 6**). Some joints, especially the hips and spinal joints, can be very hard to visualize on radiography. Where lesions in these joints are suspected, a computed tomography scan is more sensitive

Table 2
Neoplasia reported in raptor species in veterinary literature.

Tumor	Species	Sites
Fibrosarcoma	Many	Many sites described Described as locally invasive with metastatic potential
Myxofibroma	Cape griffon vulture (Gyps coprotheres)	Locally invasive on plantar foot
Fibroma	European kestrel (Falco tinnunculus)	Firm masses with predilection for skin/subcutaneous tissues of wing, leg, face, beak, neck or sternum
Histiocytic sarcoma	Great horned owl (Bubo virginianus)	Multicentric distribution Large highly pleomorphic tumors
Lipoma	Northern goshawk (accipiter gentilis), American kestrel (Falco sparvarius), Saker falcon (Falco cherrug), Gyr falcon (Falco rusticolis) Great-horned owl (Bubo virginianus)	Sites included feet, dorsal wing and adjacent to preen gland Rarely reported in raptors, which is surprising given frequent obesity problems This author has seen a single liposarcoma case in an aged Lugger falcon (Falco jugger) with metastases in the liver
Osteosarcoma	Hybrid falcon, Eurasian buzzard (Buteo buteo)	Sites on radius and sternum. Slow growing but destructive
Osteoma/chondroma	European kestrel (Falco tinnunculus) and multiple owls.	Sites include radius, frontal bone and tibiotarsus
Rhabdomyosarcoma	Lappet faced vulture (Torgos tracheliotus)	Myocardium
Leiomyoma	Golden eagle (Aquila chrysaetos), Peregrine falcon (Falco peregrinus)	Digit of foot; liver
Mixed cell tumor	Seychelles kestrel (Falco ararea)	Multiple lesions were found on the chest and head Tumor showed a mixture of tissues, including lymphangiomatous, epithelial, and chondromatous
Adenocarcinoma	Gypaetus barbatus, Buteo buteo, Buteo jamaicensis, Hieraaetus ayresii, falco peregrinus, falco punctatus, falco columbarius, Falco biarmicus, Aquila chrysaetos, Accipiter gentilis, Athene noctua, Bubo virgianus	Multiple primary and secondary sites

Adenoma	Hybrid falcon, Long crested eagle (*Lophaetus occipitalis*) and red tailed hawk (*Buteo jamaicensis*) Cinereous vulture (*Aegypius monarchus*)	Nasolacrimal duct and kidney
Cystadenocarcinoma	Peregrine falcon (*Falco peregrinus*)	Ovary
Carcinoma	Merlin (*Falco columbarius*), Red tailed hawk (*Buteo jamaicensis*), Augur buzzard (*Buteo augur*)	These aggressive neoplasms (some with marked necrosis) were found in kidney and air sac with secondary tumors in the liver
Cholangiocarcinoma	Red-tailed hawk (*Buteo jamaicensis*) Golden eagle (*A chrysaetos*)	Liver with multiple secondaries including femur
Bile duct carcinoma	Northern goshawk (*Accipiter gentilis*); Red-tailed hawk (*Buteo jamiacensis*); Golden eagle (*A chrysaetos*)	Liver with multiple metastases
Thyroid follicular cystadenoma/ thyroid cystic fibroadenoma/ thyroid follicular carcinoma	Crested cara cara (*Polyborus plancus*), Black chested buzzard eagle (*Geranoaetus melanoleucus*), Barred owl (*Strix varia*)	Tumors showed benign proliferation of thyroid follicles The carcinoma in the Barred owl was associated with raised thyroid hormone levels
Adrenal cortical carcinoma	Long crested eagle (*L occipitalis*)	—
Squamous cell carcinoma	*Falco peregrinus, Falco biamicus, Circus pygarus, Buteo jamaicensis, Bubo bubo, Parabuteo unicinctus, Haliaeetus leucocephalus*	Affected sites were predominately the flank or thigh with single cases affecting the palate, the metatarsal skin, the cloaca and tail base Classed as locally invasive with potential to slowly metastasize. Ulceration of overlying skin with secondary infection is a common feature Deformation of the beak seen where related tissue is involved
Epidermoid carcinoma	Red tailed hawk (*Buteo jamaicensis*)	Pharynx and nictitating membrane
Papilloma	Peregrine falcon (*Falco peregrinus*), King vulture (*Sarcoramphus papa*), Northern Goshawk (*Accipiter gentilis*), Tawny Eagle (*Aquila rapax*), and Lanner falcon (*Falco biarmicus*)	Sites include crop, glottis, cloaca and digit Lesions are proliferative often with fibrovascular stalks Unlike parrots does not seem to be viral-associated in raptors
Hemangioma	Peregrine falcon (*Falco peregrinus*)	Skin of dorsal cranium
Mast cell tumor	Burrowing owl (*Athene cucicularia*), Great horned owl (*Bubo bubo*), Short eared owl (*Asio flammeus*)	Lesions limited to oral cavity and head

(continued on next page)

Table 2
(continued)

Tumor	Species	Sites
Melanoma	Great horned owl (*Bubo virginianus*), Striped owl (*Asio clamator*) Red tailed hawk (*Buteo jamaicensis*)	Premortem cases seen in the eyes, though multiple internal sites described in necropsy cases
Astrocytoma	Great horned owl (Bubo virginianus)	Brain stem
Malignant lymphoma	Peregrine falcon (*Falco peregrinus*), Gyr falcon (*Falco rusticolus*), Snowy owl (*Nyctea scandiaca*)	Lesions seen in bone marrow, lungs, liver, pericardium, kidney, spleen, small intestine, testes, and fat
Malignant thymoma	Saker falcon (*Falco cherrug*) Burrowing owl (*Athene cunicularia*)	Lesions found in lungs suggesting metastatic spread from the thymus
Lymphoid leukosis	Merlin (*Falco columbarius*), Gray kestrel (*Falco ardosiaceus*), Harris hawk (*Parabuteo unicinctus*), European eagle owl (*Bubo bubo*)	Lesions found in liver and other viscera This author has also seen a single case in a Lanner falcon (*Falco biamarcus*) with lesions in the cranial coelom and clinical signs related to pressure on the heart
Erythroblastosis	Gyr falcon (*Falco rusticolus*)	A form of erythrocytic leukemia
Myelocytomatosis	Eastern screech owl (*Megascops asio*)	Liver and spleen
Lymphoma	Harris hawk (*P unicinctus*), Great horned owl (*Bubo virinianus*), miscellaneous hawks	Tumors characterized by neoplastic lymphocytic cells infiltrating a variety of tissues including the bone marrow Immature (neoplastic) lymphocytes can be observed in the blood film Lymphoid tumors are reported as common in *Bubo* spp, especially the Great-horned owl[21]
Marek's disease (herpesvirus)	Eurasian sparrow hawk (*accipiter nissus*), Great horned owl (*Bubo virginianus*) Little owl (*Athene noctua*) All cases were free ranging	Sites included sciatic nerve, liver, spleen, kidney and pancreas
Teratoma	Eurasian buzzard (*Buteo buteo*)	Abdominal mass
Xanthoma	Eurasian buzzard (*Buteo buteo*), Bateleur (*Therathopius ecaudatus*) Merlin (*Falco columbarius*)	Sites included infraorbital sinus, abdomen, spleen and liver
Mesothelioma	Ferruginous hawk (*Buteo regalis*)	Lesions (papillomatous branching tumors) were in the triosseum, pneumatic humerus and lung

Data from refs.[21,22,25–27]

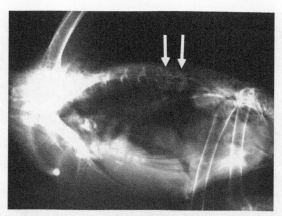

Fig. 5. Note the bony reaction at the spinal joints in this aged Common buzzard (*Buteo buteo*). Arrows indicate bony reaction at spinal joints.

(**Fig. 7**). Joint cytology may be useful to differentiate osteoarthritis from septic arthritis or gout. In terms of management of osteoarthritis, there are various methods that may be used. In all cases, regular monitoring should be carried out along with quality-of-life evaluation (discussed elsewhere in this article) to avoid welfare compromise as the condition worsens.

- Reduce joint loading.
  - ○ Sympathetic perching, with respect to shape, width, and materials all appropriate for the species and size of bird.
  - ○ Management of body weight and correct diet.
  - ○ Exercise management to decrease joint trauma and maintain mobility.
  - ○ Additional heat in aviaries in colder weather.
- Nutraceuticals and alternative therapies.

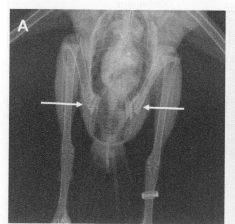
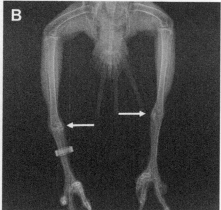

Fig. 6. (*A*) Bony proliferation and osteoarthritis of the hips in a Turkey vulture (*Cathartes aura*). Arrows indicate hip joints. (*B*) More subtle changes associated with osteoarthritis in both intertarsal joints of a Harris' hawk (*Parabuteo unicinctus*). Arrows indicate intertarsal joints.

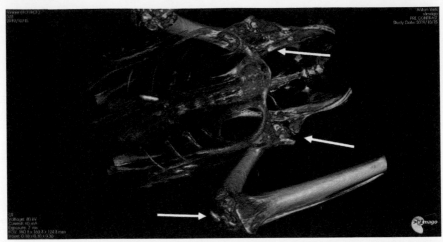

Fig. 7. Computed tomography scan showing extensive bony proliferation in the hips and stifles of an aged Hooded vulture (*Necrosyrtes monarchus*). Arrows indicate both hip joints and the left stifle.

- o Glucosamine, omega-3 polyunsaturated fatty acids, and chondroitin sulfate have been suggested as useful in management of osteoarthritis.[32] Polysulfated glycosaminoglycans have also been suggested, but have been associated with fatal coagulopathy in 2 raptors.[33]
- o Acupuncture has been described as beneficial in many species including birds.[34] Chiropractic therapy is also described as useful in birds, but should

Table 3
Analgesics for use in raptor osteoarthritis

Type of Drug	Drug	Dose Rate	Comments
Nonsteroidal anti-inflammatory drug	Meloxicam	0.5–1 mg/kg q12–24 h im/po	Rapid metabolism in Red-tailed hawks suggest more frequent dosing may be needed.
	Carprofen	1–5 mg/kg q12–24 h im/po	Higher dose rates may be effective for 24 h.
Opiate	Tramadol	5 mg/kg po bid Bald eagle 5 mg/kg po American kestrel 11 mg/kg po Red-tailed hawk	Multiple doses resulted in sedative effects. Significant antinociceptive effects for 1.5–9.0 h after administration. Higher doses well tolerated but produced little additional effect. Single dose study resulted in human plasma therapeutic concentrations for approximately 4 h.
	Gabapentin	11 mg/kg po q8 h	Great horned owls pharmacokinetic study.

Abbreviation: po, by mouth.
Data from refs.[30,36–40]

always be carried out by an experienced qualified practitioner; otherwise, harm may result.[35] Although homeopathy has also been described in birds, this author cannot recommend it and especially not as a sole therapy owing to a lack of credible evidence for its efficacy in veterinary medicine.[32]

- Analgesia – see **Table 3**.[30,36–39]
  - Nonsteroidal anti-inflammatory drugs—These are the mainstay of osteoarthritis management in raptors. Studies have shown differences between species in terms of pharmacokinetic and pharmacodynamics of these drugs, so, where possible, dose rates should be based on studies on the species being treated or as closely related as possible. Where this is not possible, dosage should be based on the lower end of the suggested range and titrated upwards as necessary. Regular monitoring of renal function should be carried out. In Old World Vultures, nonsteroidal anti-inflammatory drugs should be used with very great care and only meloxicam is currently recommended.[41]
  - Opiates—Tramadol has been evaluated in raptor species and did show analgesic effect in American kestrels, although the effects were short lasting. Multiple dosing in Bald eagles produced sedative effects.[39]
  - Gabapentin may be of use in some cases especially where there is neuropathic pain.[38]

LIVER AND KIDNEY DISEASE

It would be expected to see increasing likelihood of hepatic or renal failure in aging raptors, just as in other species. Neoplasia of either organ may be seen, although, as described elsewhere in this article, such cases are uncommon. Renal disease does seem to be increasingly common as birds age, although hepatic disease does not.[20] A component of this may be that of reduced presentation owing to reduced observation levels, and older birds may not always be presented for post mortem examination (died of old age).

Other than Old World Vultures, long-term use of nonsteroidal anti-inflammatory drugs do not seemed to be linked to renal disease,[42] although the cause of renal failure may often be difficult to determine on post mortem examination because primary lesions may be obscured by secondary gout deposition.

Diagnosis of renal disease is not easy in raptors.[20] Clinically, birds may seem to be well until disease is advanced. Clinical signs generally are nebulous and include weight loss, decrease activity, and decrease appetite—all difficult to detect in an

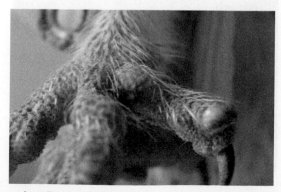

Fig. 8. Articular gout in a Barn owl (*Tyto alba*).

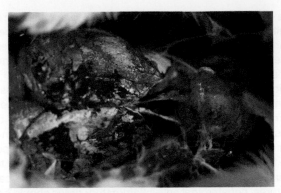

Fig. 9. Visceral gout at post mortem examination in an Old-World Vulture.

aviary bird without regular invasive monitoring. Polyuria may be seen but, again, is not easily detected unless mutes (combined fecal/urine matter) are regularly cleaned away, allowing observation of more recent muting. Polydipsia may also be a clinical sign of renal disease and any increase in drinking should signal the need to assess renal function. Gout deposition may also occur in renal failure. Articular gout is seen but is relatively uncommon (**Fig. 8**) Visceral gout is certainly seen regularly, but is usually a cause of sudden death with few premortem clinical signs (**Fig. 9**).

Blood sampling (after a 24-hour starve) may show an increase in uric acid. Urea and creatinine are not reliable analytically as they will only tend to increase in terminal renal disease. Phosphate and electrolyte changes are similarly unreliable as screening tests for renal disease.[43] Radiography may show renomegaly. Endoscopy allows observation of renal size and shape as well as permitting biopsy to assess underlying causes (**Fig. 10**).

Hepatic failure in the older bird is very often more a result of the husbandry rather than directly age related. Hepatic lipidosis is extremely common reflecting overfeeding coupled with decreased exercise. Hepatic amyloidosis[20] is also common and may

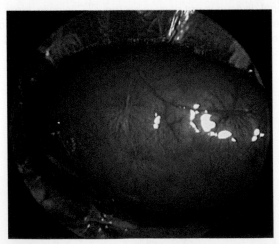

Fig. 10. Normal endoscopic appearance of the cranial pole of the left kidney in a Brown Wood owl *Strix leptogrammica*.

reflect underlying chronic inflammatory disease (eg, bumblefoot) that has not been observed or treated. Clinical signs are similar to those of renal failure, although polyuria and polydipsia are uncommon, and biliverdinuria may be seen in hepatic disease; again, regular observation of fresh urates is required to detect this. Blood sampling may detect raised liver enzymes (aspartate transaminase, glutamate dehydrogenase) or bile acids. As with renal testing, this testing is best done on a starved sample, which also allows an assessment of triglyceride and cholesterol levels without interference of postprandial effects. An increase in either of these parameters would increase concerns for hepatic lipidosis.

Radiography may indicate hepatomegaly. Ultrasound imaging gives good detail of hepatic structure and may permit guided fine-needle biopsy. Endoscopy allows direct inspection and, again, permits biopsy to assess underlying causes (**Fig. 11**).

NEUROLOGIC DISEASE AND SPECIAL SENSES

Age-related cognitive dysfunction is described by Tristan (2010),[22] but is difficult to assess, diagnose, or treat (although, anecdotally, propentofylline has been used at 5 mg/kg every 12 hours by mouth). In some cases, however, similar signs of slowing

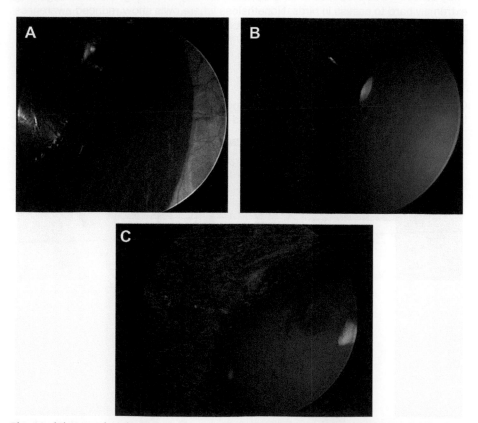

Fig. 11. (*A*) Normal endoscopic appearance of the liver in an African White-backed vulture (*Gyps africanus*). (*B*) Small bacterial abscesses in the liver of an aged African Fish eagle (*Haliaeetus vocifer*) and (*C*) the same bird after endoscopic biopsy of a lesion showing minimal hemorrhage.

and reduced awareness and reduced or altered responses may be induced by degeneration of the organs of special sense.

Neoplasia is seen but is unusual.

Ocular disease, especially cataract formation, is common in the older bird.[41] Traumatic eye lesions are also seen following "night fright" in an aviary or as a result of "clumsy" falls in arthritic birds. The most common causes of cataract formation are senile change or traumatic origin, although metabolic or inflammatory cataract may also be seen. Ocular lesions may be hard to detect unless the bird is closely inspected on a regular basis, although general observation plays a major part in the initial detection of potential problems. A bird that is reluctant to fly, crashes into objects, or misses landing perches may have reduced vision. In some cases birds may hide a unilateral lesion by only turning the good side to an observer. This behavior, again, should indicate a full ocular examination. By preference, this should be performed under anesthesia allowing full assessment of posterior and anterior segments.

Where indicated by obviously compromised vision, removal by phacoemulsification is the treatment of choice for senile cataracts. Where there is extensive ocular damage or neoplasia, then enucleation may be indicated (**Fig. 12**). Although most raptors do rely on sight as their primary sense, some nocturnal hunters use hearing as their primary sense.[44] This sense, as in other species, is likely to undergo senile change. It is extremely hard to assess in birds. Nonetheless where owls show reduced awareness or panic/surprise on approach with no obvious ocular defects, then hearing loss may be considered as a possibility.

CARDIAC DISEASE AND ATHEROSCLEROSIS

Cardiovascular disease is common in the aged raptor.[20,22] Atherosclerosis is particularly common and is likely linked to diet and reduced exercise. However, myocardial

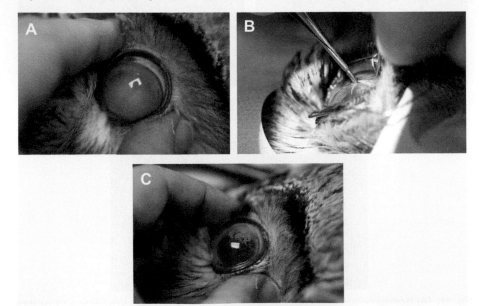

Fig. 12. (*A*) Cataract formation in a Bengalese eagle owl (*Bubo bengalensis*). (*B*) Phacoemulsification surgery in the same bird. (*C*) Postoperative view of the same eye after reinflation of the globe.

disease and aneurysms are also seen. Often there are no clinical signs with sudden death being seen.

In the flying bird, decreased exercise tolerance may be an early sign of cardiovascular disease. However, such disease can be very hard to detect in the aviary bird as there is restricted exercise capacity. Clinical signs otherwise may be nebulous and nonspecific with decreased appetite, weakness, lethargy, and decreased responsiveness. In advanced cases, collapse and/or seizures may be seen. Dyspnea is unusual. In some cases, extremities may be cold and the feet may swell.

Hepatic and/or renal disease may be seen in conjunction with cardiovascular disease and may relate to secondary congestion of these organs. For this reason, hematology and biochemistry should be assessed in cardiac cases.

Diagnostically, heart murmurs and/or dysrhythmias may be detected on auscultation, although this is not always the case and auscultation is not a sensitive means of diagnosis owing to the rapid heart rate of raptors, and the common cardiovascular diseases not primarily affecting valves to induce a murmur. In congestive cases, ascites may be seen.

Imaging may show cardiomegaly and, in atherosclerosis, thickened great vessels (**Fig. 13**). Ultrasound imaging will give better detail of heart structure as well as allowing detail of contractility and blood flow. It will also allow differentiation of cardiomegaly from pericardial effusion (**Fig. 14**). Normal radiographic and ultrasound parameters for different raptor species are being determined and some extrapolation between similar sized related species may be possible.[45,46]

Where there is a dysrhythmia, electrocardiography is indicated. Normal values are provided by Tristam (2010).[22] All cardiovascular disease carries a guarded to poor prognosis and owners should be aware of this as management of such cases may be difficult. Where therapy is warranted, the following may be used[30,36,47]:

- Diuresis—Furosemide at 0.1 to 6.0 mg/kg by mouth every 6 to 24 hours

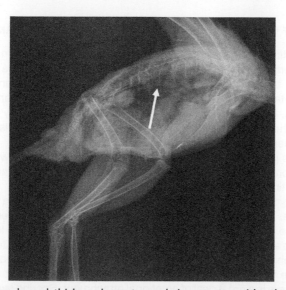

Fig. 13. Cardiomegaly and thickened great vessels in a raptor with atherosclerosis. Note that, in trained falcons, the heart will often be comparatively large and the great vessels can sometimes seem to be more prominent in the absence of internal fat deposits. This bird was a retired aviary bird and so the radiographic findings are significant. Arrow indicates thickened aorta.

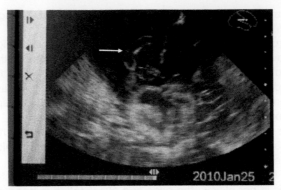

Fig. 14. Ultrasound appearance of hyperechoic thickened great vessels in a case of atherosclerosis. Arrow indicates hyperechoic thickened great vessel.

- ACE inhibitors—Enalapril (1.25 mg/kg by mouth every 12 hours) or benazepril (0.5 mg/kg by mouth every 12 hours) may be used to improve tissue and organ perfusion and may be particularly useful in cases of concurrent renal failure or where there is syncope.
- Pimobendan—This agent may be used at 0.25 mg/kg every 12 hours by mouth in cases where increased cardiac contractility is required.
- Dietary change—particularly in atherosclerosis cases. Jones[26] (2008) recommends a starve day once a week for aviary birds. Otherwise food intake should be controlled as per flying birds with daily assessment of body weight and condition.
- Antidysrhythmics[47] may be used as indicated by electrocardiography findings, although such drugs are poorly studied in raptors.

MONITORING OF QUALITY OF LIFE AND EUTHANASIA DECISION MAKING

Given the potential deficiencies in husbandry and diet resulting from reduced monitoring, it is recommended that geriatric birds should, in reality, be checked more frequently rather than less. Falconry birds are usually well-trained, and, increasingly, zoo birds are better trained. As such, birds can be trained to a perch on scales to allow regular weighing. Regular feeding on the fist allows checking of body condition and a basic physical check. This practice will enable earlier detection of disease as well as better management of bodyweight and reduced obesity.

Where there is preexisting disease, more intensive management will enable better assessment of progress of disease and therefore better decision making regarding medication and timing of euthanasia in severe cases.

A useful tool in older animals with slowly progressive conditions is a scoring method for quality of life. Arthritic cases, in particular, are usefully monitored using scoring because it can be hard in birds (that hide signs of pain) to assess pain levels and hence when to increase analgesia, or when to euthanize (Please see Dan H. Johnson's article, "Geriatric Hedgehogs," in this issue for humane techniques of euthanasia in exotic animals). In both the zoo and falconry situations, there can be reluctance to euthanize older birds to whom there is a great deal of emotional attachment. Scoring systems can make these decisions simpler and achieve better compliance with keeping staff.

There is no generic scoring system for these birds and it is generally best to draw up plans on an individual basis. The importance is to achieve consistency between scorers and, where there is a single keeper (and more potential for attachment and bias in scoring) a regular oversight from an independent scorer. Factors that may be considered in development of a scoring system should include:

- Appetite
- Body weight
- Body condition
- Activity levels, including
  - Use of perches
  - Movement between perches, amount of movement, speed of movement, manner of movement
  - Speed of movement between perches, and approaching food trays/keeper
  - For leg joints
    - Loading of weight on each leg (always standing on 1 leg?)
    - Strength of grip
    - Lameness when walking
    - Bumblefoot lesions (can be graded as per Bailey [2008])[48]
  - For wing joints
    - Drooping wings
    - Ability to fly/length of flights
    - Ability to extend wings

Veterinary involvement should also be considered a part of geriatric raptor management. It is common practice in falconry to have veterinary checks before and after the hunting season, yet these are often not performed for the retired aviary bird. The veterinary examination performed on a regular basis is another means of providing an independent assessment of quality of life, in particular in detection of early stage disease. Coupled with examination, regular blood sampling (for hematology and liver/kidney function as minimum) should also be considered, especially if on long-term analgesia. An important consideration is that raptors should always be starved for 24 hours before such checks and sampling to avoid confusion with postprandial increases in uric acid, triglycerides, and cholesterol.

DISCLOSURE

The author declares that, other than being a practicing clinician working with raptors, he has no competing interests with any matter raised in this article.

REFERENCES

1. del Hoyo J, Elliott A, Sargatal J. Handbook of the birds of the world volume 2: new world vultures to Guineafowl. Barcelona (Spain): Lynx Edicions; 1994.
2. del Hoyo J, Elliott A, Sargatal J. Handbook of the birds of the world volume 5: Barn-owls to hummingbirds. Barcelona (Spain): Lynx Edicions; 1999.
3. Fox N. Understanding the bird of prey. Blaine (WA): Hancock House Publishers; 1995.
4. Parry-Jones JF. Care, captive breeding and conservation. Newton Abbott (United Kingdom): David & Charles; 1988.
5. Cooper JE. Birds of prey, health & disease. 3rd edition. Oxford (United Kingdom): Blackwell Science; 2002.
6. Available at: https://ich.unesco.org/en/lists.

7. Olendorff SE, Oldendorff R. An extensive bibliography on falconry: eagles, hawks, falcons and other diurnal birds of prey, vols. 1-3. USA: R. Oldendorff, Publisher; 1968-1970.

8. Salvin FH, Brodrick W. Falconry in the British Isles. London: John Van Voorst; 1855.

9. Dalton B. The passage falcon. Fair Oak (United Kingdom): Falcon Leisure Publishing; 2015.

10. Heidenreich M. Birds of prey medicine and management. Oxford (United Kingdom): Blackwell Science; 1997.

11. Olney P, Schmidt CR, Lint KC. Longevity of birds of prey and owls in captivity. In: Lucas J, editor. International zoo yearbook 10. Zoological Society of London; 1970. p. 36–7.

12. Minnemann D, Busse H. Longevity of birds of prey and owls at East Berlin Zoo. In: Olney PJS, editor. International zoo yearbook 23. Zoological Society of London; 1984. p. 108–10.

13. British Trust for Ornithology Longevity Records. Available at: https://app.bto.org/ring/countyrec/results2018/longevity.htm.

14. USGS Longevity Records. Available at: https://www.pwrc.usgs.gov/bbl/longevity/longevity_main.cfm.

15. Euring Longevity Records. Available at: https://euring.org/data-and-codes/longevity-list.

16. Brown L, Amadon D. Eagles, hawks & falcons of the world. Secaucus (NJ): Wellfleet Press; 1989.

17. Baker K. Identification Guide to European non-passerines; BTO Guide 24. Thetford (United Kingdom): British Trust for Ornithology; 1993.

18. Warren K, Le Souef A, Cooey C, et al. Diagnostic Testing of Age of Birds and Its Applications. In: Speer BL, editor. Current therapy in avian medicine and surgery. St Louis (MO): Elsevier; 2016. p. 527–30.

19. Parry-Jones J. Raptor husbandry and falconry techniques. In: Chitty J, Lierz M, editors. BSAVA manual of raptors, pigeons and passerine birds. Gloucester (United Kingdom): BSAVA; 2008. p. 7–13.

20. Chitty J, Lierz M, editors. BSAVA manual of raptors, pigeons and passerine birds. Gloucester (United Kingdom): BSAVA; 2008. p. 7–13.

21. Beaufrere H, Laniesse D. Medicine of Strigiformes. In: Speer BL, editor. Current therapy in avian medicine and surgery. St Louis (MO): Elsevier; 2016. p. 566–81.

22. Tristram T. The aging raptor. Vet Clin North Am Exot Anim Pract 2010;13:51–84.

23. Chitty J. Postmortem findings in a Collection of Captive Raptors. ExoticsCon Proceedings. St Louis, MI, September 29 – October 3, 2019. p. 124–5.

24. Chitty J. Pyoderma and squamous cell carcinoma in Harris' hawks. Proceedings of the 1st international Conference on Avian, Herpetological, & Exotic Animal Medicine. Wiesbaden, Germany, April 20 – 26, 2013. p. 374–5.

25. Forbes NA, Cooper JE, Higgins RJ. Neoplasms of birds of prey. In: Lumeij JT, Remple D, Redig PT, et al, editors. Raptor biomedicine III. Lake Worth (FL): Zoological Education Network; 2000.

26. Jones R. Raptors: systemic and non-infectious disorders. In: Chitty J, Lierz M, editors. BSAVA manual of raptors, pigeons and passerine birds. Gloucester(United Kingdom): BSAVA; 2008. p. 284–98.

27. Montijano MG, Lopez IL, Eiguran AA, et al. Cystadenocarcinoma and leiomyoma in a peregrine falcon (Falcon peregrinus brookei). Vet Rec 2008;162:859–61.

28. Exotic species cancer research alliance. Available at: https://web.stanford.edu/group/bustamante_lab/cgi-bin/ESCRA/.

29. Zehnder A, Graham J, Antonissen G. Update on cancer treatment in exotics. Vet Clin North Am Exot Anim Pract 2018;21:465–509.
30. Meredith A, editor. BSAVA Small animal formulary 9th edition- Part B: exotic pets. Gloucester (United Kingdom): BSAVA; 2015.
31. Doneley B. Avian medicine and surgery in practice: companion and avian birds. 2nd Edition. Boca Raton (FL): CRC Press; 2016.
32. Ness RD. Integrative therapies. In: Harrison G, Lightfoot T, editors. Clinical avian medicine. Lake Worth (FL): Zoological Education Network; 2006. p. 343–64.
33. Anderson K, Garner MM, Reed HH, et al. Hemorrhagic diathesis in avian species following intramuscular administration of polysulfated glycosaminoglycan. J Zoo Wildl Med 2013;44(1):93–9.
34. Koski MA. Acupuncture for zoological companion animals. Vet Clin North Am Exot Anim Pract 2011;14:141–54.
35. Marziani JA. Nontraditional therapies (traditional Chinese medicine and Chiropractic) in exotic animals. Vet Clin North Am Exot Anim Pract 2018;21:511–28.
36. Carpenter JW. Exotic animal formulary. 5th Edition. St Louis (MO): Elsevier; 2018.
37. Balko JA, Chinnadurai SK. Advancements in evidence-based analgesia in exotic animals. Vet Clin North Am Exot Anim Pract 2017;20:899–915.
38. Hawkins MG, Paul-Murphy J. Avian analgesia. Vet Clin North Am Exot Anim Pract 2011;14:61–80.
39. Souza MJ, Cox SK. Tramadol use in zoologic medicine. Vet Clin North Am Exot Anim Pract 2011;14:117–30.
40. Naidoo V, Wolter K, Cromarty AD, et al. The pharmacokinetics of meloxicam in vultures. J Vet Pharmacol Ther 2008;31(2):128–34.
41. Williams DL. Raptors; ophthalmology. In: Chitty J, Lierz M, editors. BSAVA manual of raptors, pigeons and passerine birds. Gloucester(United Kingdom): BSAVA; 2008. p. 278–83.
42. Swarup DP, Patra RC, Prakash V, et al. Safety of meloxicam to critically endangered Gyps vultures and other scavenging birds in India. Anim Conservat 2007 May;10:192–8.
43. Lumeij JT. Pathophysiology diagnosis and treatment of renal disorders in birds of prey. In: Lumeij JT, Remple JD, Redig PT, et al, editors. Raptor biomedicine III. Lake worth (FL): Zoological Education Network; 2000. p. 169–78.
44. Dooling RJ, Lohr B, Dent ML. Hearing in birds and reptiles. In: Dooling RJ, Fay RR, Popper AN, editors. Comparative hearing: birds and reptiles. New York: Springer-Verlag; 2000. p. 308–60.
45. Barbon AR, Smith S, Forbes N. Radiographic evaluation of cardiac size in four falconiform species. J Avian Med Surg 2010;24(3):222–7.
46. Pees M, Krautwald-Junghanns ME. Cardiovascular physiology and diseases of pet birds. Vet Clin North Am Exot Anim Pract 2009;12(1):81–97.
47. Fitzgerald BC, Dias S, Martorell J. Cardiovascular drugs in avian, small mammal and reptile medicine. Vet Clin North Am Exot Anim Pract 2018;21:399–442.
48. Bailey T, Lloyd C. Raptors: disorders of the feet. In: Chitty, Lierz, editors. BSAVA Manual of Raptors, Pigeons and Passerine Birds. Uk: BSAVA: Gloucester; 2008. p. 176–89.

Selected Veterinary Concerns of Geriatric Rats, Mice, Hamsters, and Gerbils

Michael Dutton, DVM, MS, DABVP (Canine & Feline Practice), DABVP (Avian Practice), DABVP (Exotic Companion Mammal Practice), DABVP (Reptile & Amphibian Practice)

KEYWORDS

- Rat • Mouse • Gerbil • Hamster • Geriatric • Nutrition • Euthanasia • Pain

KEY POINTS

- Due to improvements in husbandry and increased availability of veterinary specialists, more geriatric rats, mice, hamsters, and gerbils with associated aged pet diseases are being seen by veterinarians.
- Given the short life span of these pets, quality-of-life concerns should be discussed with owners as part of the overall veterinary medical plan.
- Many of the typical dog and cat formulary drugs can be used in these geriatric pets with minimal modifications.

INTRODUCTION

Improved husbandry and better knowledge of exotic pets have led to a gradual increase in the life span of pets, such as rats, mice, hamsters, and gerbils. Much of the information on these senior patients is derived from the laboratory animal studies and anecdotal practitioner information.

Although the small size of some of the patients makes blood collection problematic for hematology and biochemical function testing, the advent of polymerase chain reaction testing (**Box 1**) and other molecular diagnostics is allowing practitioners to test for specific etiologies with the very small biologic samples available. Both ultrasonography (**Figs. 1 and 2**) and radiology (**Figs. 3–5**) also are valuable diagnostic modalities.

GENERAL CONCERNS FOR GERIATRIC RATS, MICE, HAMSTERS, AND GERBILS
Aging Changes

The species outlined in this article have relatively short lives and reach geriatric status in a matter of a 2 years to 5 years. Although clients intellectually know this, it can be a

Exotic and Bird Clinic of New England, c/o Weare Animal Hospital, 91 North Stark Highway, Weare, NH 03281, USA
E-mail address: mdutton@weareanimalhospital.com

Vet Clin Exot Anim 23 (2020) 525–548
https://doi.org/10.1016/j.cvex.2020.04.001
1094-9194/20/© 2020 Elsevier Inc. All rights reserved.
vetexotic.theclinics.com

Box 1
Partial list of polymerase chain reaction tests available for rats, mice, hamsters, and gerbils

Aspiculuris tetraptera

Coccidia

Ectromelia

Epizootic diarrhea of infant mice

Encephalomyocarditis virus

Fur mites

Hantavirus

Helicobacter species

K virus

Lactate dehydrogenase–elevating virus

Leptospira

Lymphocytic choriomeningitis virus

Mites

Mouse adenoviruses type 1 and type 2

Mouse cytomegaloviruses type 1 and type 2

Mouse hepatitis

Mouse minute virus

Mouse norovirus

Mouse parvovirus

Mouse polyomavirus

Mousepox virus

Mouse rotavirus

Mycoplasma species

Pasteurella multocida

Pinworms

Pneumocystis carinii

Pneumonia virus of mice

Rat-bite fever

Rat coronavirus

Reovirus type 3

Rodent infestation panel

Salmonella

Sendai virus

Seoul virus

Shigella

Sialodacryoadenitis virus

Streptobacillus moniliformis

Streptococcus pneumoniae

Syphacia muris

Syphasia obvelata

Theiler murine encephalomyelitis virus

Tick-borne encephalitis virus

Tyzzer disease

Yersinia pestis

Yersinia pseudotuberculosis

surprise to them when discussing kidney disease or osteoarthritis, when a pet may be only 18 months old.

The aging changes seen in these species mimic similar changes in the more common species, such as dogs and cats. Changes, such as sleeping more, moving less, decreased interaction with owners, and so forth, are common. Miscellaneous skin masses appear with some regularity and weight gain may occur.

These species have continually growing incisors that may need periodic grinding if malocclusion has occurred (**Fig. 6**).

Nutrition

There is little information about dietary changes that may be needed for these species. In general, the dietary requirements that are used for adolescence or adulthood seem appropriate for the geriatric patient.

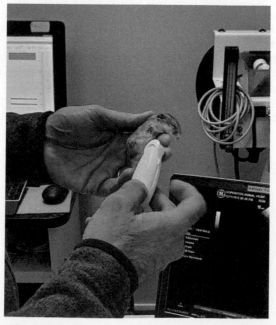

Fig. 1. Ultrasonography is an invaluable diagnostic tool. The use of a microconvex or linear probe typically is needed for these small patients.

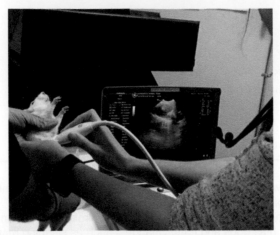

Fig. 2. Suspected mediastinal mass located on ultrasound.

Quality of Life

Knowing when a patient is not experiencing an appropriate quality of life includes weighing many factors. One proposed scale is the HHHHHMM algorithm.[1]

Hurt

The hurt criterion assesses the pain that a pet is exhibiting. Also important to acknowledge is that dyspnea also can be painful. In humans, dyspnea is ranked high as a painful process. The use of nonsteroidal anti-inflammatory drugs (NSAIDs) is warranted early in the course of pain to minimize the establishment of wind-up pain. Clients should be counseled on the signs of pain and the need to medicate for pain even when a pet may not be exhibiting signs.

Meloxicam commonly is used because it already is in a suspension form. For very small patients, it can be diluted for more appropriate dosing with the preferred diluent being methylcellulose products.

For male rats, oral tramadol (40 mg/kg, orally) and oral buprenorphine (0.5 mg/kg and 0.6 mg/kg, orally) have been shown to be effective analgesia. In female rats, oral buprenorphine was not effective but oral tramadol (20 mg/kg, 30 mg/kg, and

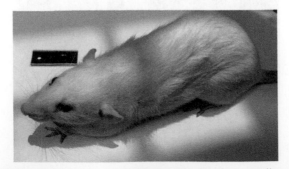

Fig. 3. Standard 2-view radiographs can be diagnostic. For these smaller patients, a dorso-ventral position can be easier to obtain than a ventrodorsal projection.

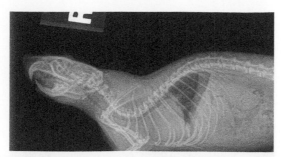

Fig. 4. Suspected cranial mediastinal mass, which was confirmed on ultrasound.

40 mg/kg) was effective.[2] Anecdotally veterinarians have used tramadol in gerbils and hamsters.

Oral gabapentin is effective in rats primarily for neuropathic pain control.[3,4] Oral gabapentin (30–100 mg/kg, orally) is effective in mice.[5] Anecdotally, veterinarians have used gabapentin in hamsters and gerbils.

Cannabidiol (CBD) is a new pharmaceutical used in veterinary medicine, but little evidence-based information is available. There are several over-the-counter CBD oils and 1 approved human medication (Epidiolex, Greenwich Biosciences, Carlsbad,

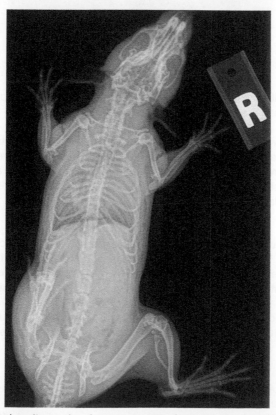

Fig. 5. Dorsoventral radiograph of same rat. In this patient, a mediastinal mass was confirmed on ultrasound.

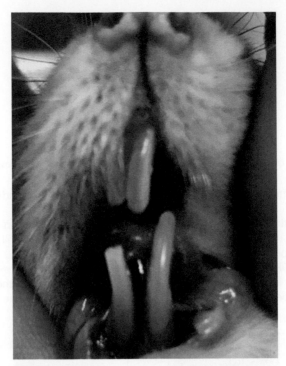

Fig. 6. Overgrown incisors on a rat.

California). As with many over-the-counter supplements, quality control may be an issue, and owners are advised to pick a brand name with third-party laboratory validation.

One study showed CBD caused liver damage in mice at the allometrically equivalent of the human maximum dose.[6] Topically applied 1% CBD gel over arthritic joints appeared to decrease inflammation in a rat arthritis model.[7] CBD in a hamster report showed that dosing of 1.25 mg/kg to 20 mg/kg, orally, protected against cerebral ischemia after bilateral carotid occlusion.[8]

Hunger

Given the continually growing natures of these pets' teeth, malocclusion or incisor overgrowth (**Fig. 7**) can lead to problems masticating and prehending food, leading to hunger and debilitation. Many times, this manifests as weight loss, more time at feed bowls but little actual consumption of food, or associated pathology, such as abscessation at the dental site. Correction of dental issues and/or force-feeding with appropriate diet items or prepackaged formulas can alleviate hunger in the short term. Some owners are able to supplement a pet's feeding habits with scheduled force-feeding.

Hydration

The hydration status of a geriatric pet can be impacted by various issues. These include metabolic diseases, such as diabetes mellitus and kidney dysfunction; dental issues, for example, where a patient cannot use a water dripper bottle appropriately; or arthritis, impacting mobility to the water system. Owners may notice apparent

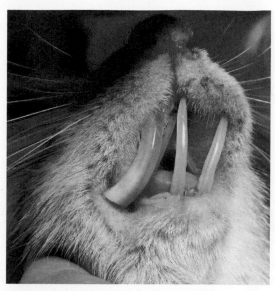

Fig. 7. Inability to prehend food can lead to hunger and debilitation.

weight loss or sunken/closed eyes on their pet. On physical examination, the standard skin turgor parameters used for measuring dehydration in other veterinary species apply to this group of patients (**Fig. 8**).

Hygiene

Pets that are in distress many times stop normal grooming and become unthrifty. Many times, owners notice the poor fur condition and that is a reason for them bringing a pet to the veterinarian. Because a majority cases of poor hygiene can be attributed to another underlying disease, the veterinarian should focus on determining the primary source of a pet's discomfort (**Fig. 9**).

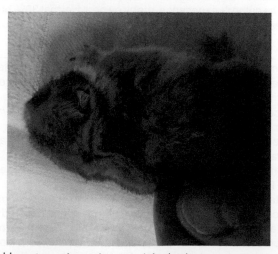

Fig. 8. Dehydrated hamster estimated at 7% dehydration.

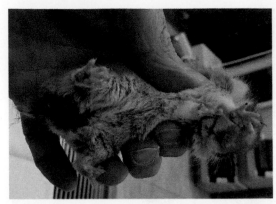

Fig. 9. Hamster with unthrifty perianal area. This patient had colitis and ultimately prolapsed 10 mm of the large intestine.

Happiness
Happiness pertains to owner and veterinarian assessment of a pet's attitude and overall well-being. If a pet seems anxious, fearful, sensitive to touch, and so forth, all are factors that can be considered in this category of happiness.

Mobility
Preemptive use of NSAIDs can prolong the pain-free mobility of these patients. As in other species, the expectation is that an NSAID will decrease in effectiveness as the disease process progresses. Pain also can result in a pet resisting handling or petting. Adding additional pain medications, such as gabapentin and tramadol, at this time may be helpful.

More good days than bad days
Geriatric pets can have waxing and waning of their condition, resulting in good days and bad days. Many owners understand this concept and a discussion about the percentages of good days and bad days can help owners understand the progression of the aging process and help owners set up their own parameters for when quality of life may be compromised. In the author's experience, many owners feel that 30% bad days is a common area where euthanasia discussion starts to occur with more frequency.

Pharmaceuticals
1. Pain management is paramount in maintaining quality of life and function. Commonly used veterinary medications can be used in rats, mice, hamsters, and gerbils (**Table 1**).[9] Opioids may cause sedation in these pets.
2. Cardiac medications can be useful for many pets in early to advanced stages of cardiovascular disease. Signs of cardiac disease are similar to other mammals and include cardiomegaly, increased interstitial pattern on radiographs, and possible pleural effusion (**Fig. 10**).
3. Common veterinary cardiac medications can be used in these species (**Table 2**).[10]
4. Supplemental feeding
   Supplemental feeding with several products is manageable for most owners. The feedings can include a pureed version of the normal pelleted food a pet consumes. Packaged products, such as Hills a/d, Oxbow Carnivore Care, and Emeraid products, are options. Depending on a pet's condition, supplemental feedings may occur daily or less frequently.

Table 1
Drugs used for pain management

Drug	Rat	Mouse	Gerbil	Hamster
Meloxicam	0.5–2.0 mg/kg, PO, SQ, q24h	1–5 mg/kg, PO, SQ, q24 h	0.5 mg/kg, PO, SQ, q24h	0.5 mg/kg, PO, SQ q24h
Carprofen	2–5 mg/kg, PO, SQ, IM, q12–24 h	2–5 mg/kg, PO, SQ, IM, q12–24h	5 mg/kg, SQ, q24h	5 mg/kg, SQ, q24h
Butorphanol	1–2 mg/kg, SQ, IM, IV, q2–4h	1–2 mg/kg, SQ, IP, q2-4h	1–5 mg/kg, SQ, q4h	1–5 mg/kg, SQ, q4h
Buprenorphine	0.05–0.1 mg/kg, SQ, IM, q6-12h	0.05–0.1 mg/kg, SQ, q6-12h	0.1–0.2 mg/kg, SQ, q8h	0.5 mg/kg, SQ, q8h
Tramadol	5–20 mg/kg, PO, SQ, IV, IP	5–40 mg/kg, SQ, IP	5–10 mg/kg, PO, q12–24h	5–10 mg/kg, PO, q12–24h
Gabapentin	50 mg/kg, PO, q24h	10–70 mg/kg, PO, q24h	50 mg/kg, PO, q24h	50 mg/kg, PO, q24h
Ketoprofen	2–5 mg/kg, SC, IM, q12–24h	2–5 mg/kg, SC, IM, q12–24h	5 mg/kg, SQ, q24h	5 mg/kg, SQ, q24h

5. Directed therapies

Depending on the etiology of the geriatric pet's condition, there may be specific therapeutic interventions that can occur. These include subcutaneous fluid administration, antibiotics for any bacterial infection (such as from dental disease), surgical removal of benign and malignant neoplasia, cardiac medications, blood pressure modulators, and hormonal medications.

Dental Issues

Dental issues are common, and special attention needs to be placed on treating concerns, such as overgrown incisors. An owner may note decreased eating habits (and concurrent decrease in fecal matter), and a physical examination usually reveals a dental malocclusion or overgrowth (**Figs. 11** and **12**).

Therapy usually is the grinding down of the offending overgrown tooth, and treatment of any concurrent skin abscess and management of pain. The use of nail

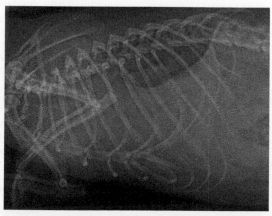

Fig. 10. Pleural effusion in a rat secondary to congestive heart failure.

Table 2
Drugs used for cardiovascular disease

Species	Drug	Dosage	Comments, Indication
Therapeutics for Use in Small Exotic Mammals with Cardiovascular Disease			
Hamster	Amlodipine	10 mg/kg/d in food	Calcium antagonist Amlodipine prevents cell death and fibrosis and reduces cardiac dysfunction in cardiomyopathic hamsters.
Rat	Atenolol	5 mg/kg	β-blocker, hypertrophic cardiomyopathy Prolongs filling, decreases myocardial ischemia
Hamster	Digoxin	0.05–0.01 mg/kg, PO, q12–24h	Positive inotrope Right-sided heart failure, nonresponsive cardiomyopathy, dilated cardiomyopathy Also indicated for atrial fibrillation
Hamster	Diltiazem	25 mg/kg/d, PO	Calcium channel blocker Benzodiazepine like calcium antagonist Increases ventricular filling, reduces heart rate and blood pressure; reduces myocardial oxygen consumption
Hamster	Enalapril	0.5 mg/kg PO, q24–48h, 20 mg/kg/d in food	Angiotensin-converting enzyme inhibitor Balanced vasodilator; avoid use in animal with concurrent renal disease.
Hamster, mouse, rat	Furosemide	1–10 mg/kg IM, SQ, PO, q4–12h	Diuretic, reduction of ascites, pleural effusion, pulmonary edema
Rodents in general	Isoprenaline	0.1–1 mg/kg/min IV, IC Total dose 5–10 μg/kg	Complete heart block, low cardiac output
All	Nitroglycerin ointment 2%	1/16 in/kg Apply to hairless region q12–24h	Initial adjunctive venodilation for emergency use
Rodents	Propranolol	0.1 mg/kg IV, IC	β-blocker, hypertrophic cardiomyopathy Prolongs filling, decreases myocardial ischemia Tachyarrhythmia
Rat	Pimobendan	1 mg/kg	Phosphodiesterase inhibitor (which causes peripheral ateriodilation and venodilation and improved myocardial contractility)
All	Omega 3	25 mg/d	Generally recommended nutraceuticals for cardiac support in rodents and small exotic mammals
All	Oils, including flax oil	10–30 mg/d	Generally recommended nutraceuticals for cardiac support in rodents and small exotic mammals

(continued on next page)

Table 2
(*continued*)

Therapeutics for Use in Small Exotic Mammals with Cardiovascular Disease			
Species	Drug	Dosage	Comments, Indication
	Coenzyme Q10	25 mg/d	Generally recommended nutraceuticals for cardiac support in rodents and small exotic mammals
	L-carnitine	50 mg/d	Generally recommended nutraceuticals for cardiac support in rodents and small exotic mammals
All	Taurine	50 mg/d	Generally recommended nutraceuticals for cardiac support in rodents and small exotic mammals
Hamster, rat	Verapamil	0.25–0.5 mg/hamster SQ, 5 mg/kg/d IP, 0.75 mg/mL in drinking water	Calcium channel blocker Increases ventricular filling, reduces heart rate and blood pressure, reduces myocardial oxygen consumption

clippers to clip teeth short can lead to fracturing of the enamel and dentin, with extension into the root, leading to pain and infection. For this reason, pets should be anesthetized and teeth ground and shaped to proper length and position with low-speed dental burs. Equipment is readily available from veterinary distributors **(Fig. 13)**.

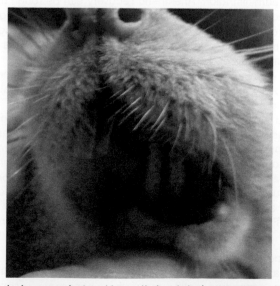

Fig. 11. The upper incisors are deviated laterally but it is the overgrown lower incisors that are the primary reason this rat cannot eat.

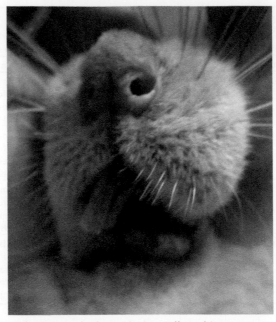

Fig. 12. Significant reduction in the lower incisors allow this rat to eat normally.

Anesthesia

Contemporary anesthetics and methods minimize, but do not eliminate, anesthetic risk for surgical intervention.

1. Alfaxalone is a neurosteroid anesthetic that is short acting and has the benefit of intramuscular administration. Anesthetic recovery can be rough unless other pre-anesthetic medications, such as an opioid, are used. It can sting upon injection. Dosing has been reported as 20 mg/kg, intramuscularly, or 120 mg/kg, intraperitoneally (IP), for rodents.[11] Anecdotally, practitioners have used this subcutaneously and for pre-euthanasia sedation.
2. Propofol is a γ-aminobutyric acid inhibitory short-acting anesthetic that can be used intravenously (IV) at a dose of 7.5 mg/kg to 10 mg/kg (rats) or 12 mg/kg to 26 mg/kg (mice).[11]
3. Isoflurane and sevoflurane can be used with an anesthetic cone or induction chamber. These are short-acting gas anesthetics. Recovery can be rough and the use of a preanesthetic medications, such as an opioid, is recommended. If possible, endotracheal intubation should be performed but, given the size of these pets, that may not be doable. Supraglottic devices have been constructed and used successfully.[12] Details on construction are available online.[13] Commercially available devices are available although they may be too large for smaller pets (**Figs. 14** and **15**; v-gel: http://docsinnovent.com/products/product/rabbit-v-gel).

The author finds that a preanesthetic body radiograph can help determine whether overt cardiomegaly is present, indicating overt heart disease. Although the anesthesia procedure still may be necessary, appropriate client communications can occur prior to the anesthesia. A standard orthogonal

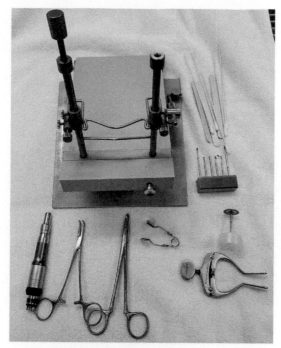

Fig. 13. Typical dental equipment employed in the author's practice.

radiograph of the thorax (and many times the whole body) typically suffices (**Figs. 16** and **17**).

Euthanasia

Unfortunately for many smaller patients, direct venous access is not possible, making IV injection of euthanasia solution improbable. Discussing options with owners about route of administration may be prudent. Options include IV access (in some cases, a small-gauge wing-tip catheter can be used for these small patients), intraosseous administration (although pets should be anesthetized to place an intraosseous infusion catheter [**Figs. 18** and **19**] or needle), intracardiac administration (using an opioid premedication and masking patients under gas anesthesia is preferable before injection), and intrathoracic administration (same caveat as for intracardiac administration). (See End of Life Decisions: Palliative Care, Hospice, and Euthanasia for Exotic Animals, for additional information regarding American Veterinary Medical Association guidelines for humane euthanasia of pets.)

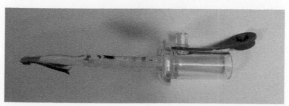

Fig. 14. Side profile of #1 v-gel. (*Courtesy of* Docsinnovent Ltd., Hempstead, UK.)

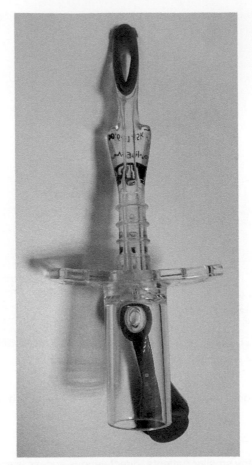

Fig. 15. Top profile of #1 v-gel. (*Courtesy of* Docsinnovent Ltd., Hempstead, UK.)

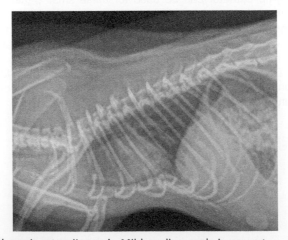

Fig. 16. Lateral thoracic rat radiograph. Mild cardiomegaly is present.

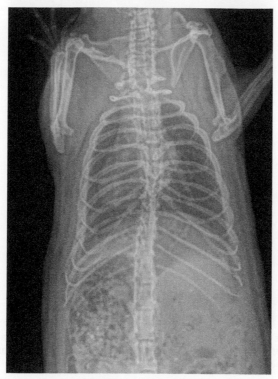

Fig. 17. Dorsoventral thoracic radiograph of same rat.

COMMON ISSUES WITH SELECTED SPECIES
Rats

The fancy rat (*Rattus norvegicus domestica*) is the most commonly kept pet rat, with most living 2 years to 3 years, although 4 years can occur. Common diseases in the geriatric rat include a variety of skin masses, multifactorial respiratory disease, mammary neoplasia, pituitary adenomas, kidney dysfunction, and neuropathies.

Multifactorial respiratory disease is the norm for rats, with a high number affected by *Mycoplasma pulmonis* coinfections. Rats usually exhibit chronic sneezing, nasal discharge, epiphora that usually is colored red to brown, and decreased appetite. Infrequently, vestibular signs may be exhibited.

There are several causes for respiratory disease, which are listed in **Table 3**.

Therapy consists of improving the environment, nutrition, use of antibiotics (enrofloxacin, 10 mg/kg, orally, every 12 h); doxycycline, 5 mg/kg, orally, every 12 h; or azithromycin (20 mg/kg, every 24 h, 7 d), and possible NSAIDs.[14] Nebulization can be beneficial. Using a nebulizer that achieves a small particle size of 3 μm is recommended, at a rate of 10 minutes to 30 minutes a session for 1 to 3 sessions a day.[15] Anecdotally, just the use of 0.9% NaCl can be beneficial for nebulization. Antibiotics, such as enrofloxacin (2–10 mg/mL saline[16]) and gentamicin (50 mg in 10 mL saline for 15 min every 8 h to 12 h[17]), can be used for nebulization.

Neoplasia is common in rats. Mammary tumors (**Figs. 20** and **21**) are easily noted by owner and clinician. Pituitary adenomas also occur commonly, but specialized imaging is required to diagnose this neoplasia.

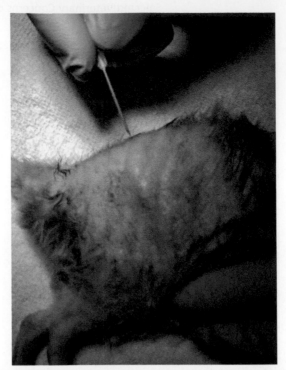

Fig. 18. Alignment of a 20-g hypodermic needle at the trochanteric fossa of the femur for an intraosseous catheter in a rat. The area is prepped and the needle advanced through the fossa and down the medullary canal.

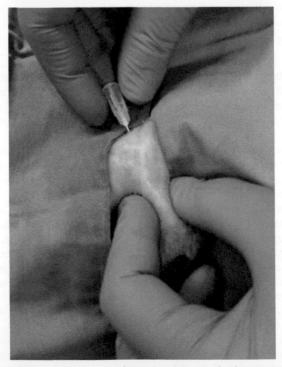

Fig. 19. Placement of the intraosseous catheter in same rat. Fluid rates equaling IV rates can be used.

Table 3	
Rat respiratory disease etiologies and risk factors	
Virus	Sendai virus
	Coronavirus
Bacteria	*Mycoplasma* spp
	Cilia-associated respiratory bacillus
	Bordetella
	Corynebacterium kutscheri
	Streptococcus spp
Environment	Poor ventilation
	Build-up of soiled bedding

Mammary tumors in female rats typically are fibroadenomas. These subcutaneous fibroadenomas can grow to 8 cm to 10 cm in diameter and the overlying skin can be

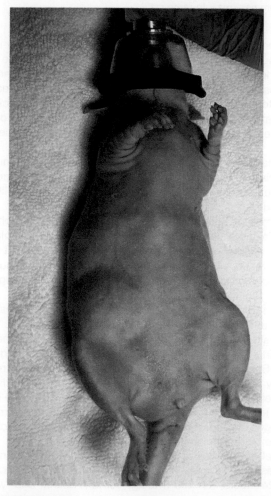

Fig. 20. Rat with mammary mass.

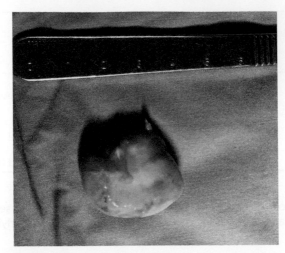

Fig. 21. Excised mammary mass in same rat.

traumatized. Mammary tumors can occur in male rats but at a lower incidence.[18] Surgical removal is recommended but other neoplasia may occur in the remaining mammary tissue. The incidence of mammary tumors, in addition to pituitary tumors, can be reduced in rats that are ovariectomized at 90 days of age compared with those that were not ovariectomized.[19] Current studies do not show a reduction in neoplasia recurrence if the rat is ovariectomized once mammary tumors have occurred. Tamoxifen, an antiestrogen compound, has been tried but liver toxicity issues have limited its use.[20]

Anecdotally, it has been used successfully to prevent further mammary fibroadenomas in rats, especially those unable to undergo ovariectomy due to comorbid disease.

In several studies, food restriction to approximately 65% of ad libitum consumed food showed a reduced incidence of mammary neoplasia.[21]

Pituitary adenomas are common in aging rats, leading to lactotroph hyperplasia and hyperprolactinemia. Increasing prolactin levels in the aged rat may play a role in mammary neoplasia development. Cabergoline, a prolactin inhibitor that suppresses pituitary prolactin secretion, can be given orally. It has been used successfully in the reducing the size of a pituitary adenoma in a rat at a dose of 0.6 mg/kg, orally, every 72 hours.[22]

As in mammary tumors, rats fed on a restricted diet had the lowest incidence of pituitary adenomas and focal pituitary hyperplasia.[23]

Chronic progressive nephrosis/nephropathy (CPN) is one of the more common causes of death in aged rats and the incidence has been reported as high as 75% in some strains (Sprague-Dawley).[24] The disease occurs more frequently in male rate and generally is of greater severity than in female rats. In CPN, lesions consist of a chronic glomerulosclerosis and interstitial disease involving the convoluted proximal tubules. The kidneys can be enlarged to twice normal size or more and are pale and mottled.[25] Signs are those seen in a renal failure state and include weight loss, lethargy, azotemia, and proteinuria.[26]

Treatment is palliative. A lower protein diet (10%–14%) is recommended and, in more severe cases, supplemental subcutaneous fluids may be necessary, dosed at 50 mL/kg, for 24 hours, to 100 mL/kg, for 24 hours, and warmed to body temperature.[27]

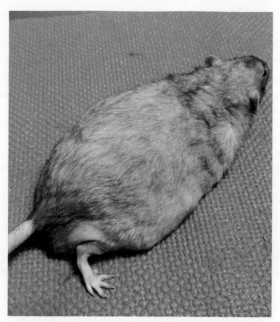

Fig. 22. This rat had progressive posterior weakness that was suspected to be radiculoneuropathy.

Posterior weakness (**Fig. 22**) or tail dragging may indicate radiculoneuropathy, with resulting disturbances in motor function. This is a degenerative disease of the spinal roots accompanied by atrophy of skeletal muscle in the lumbar region and hind limbs.[28] The incidence in rats over 24 months of age may be as high as 75% to 90%. Demyelination and vacuolation are seen in the lumbosacral roots, notably in the ventral spinal regions. Treatment with B complex, at a dose of 2 mg/kg, subcutaneously/intramuscularly, appears to decrease symptoms along with NSAIDs, such as meloxicam.[29,30]

Mice

Mammary gland adenocarcinoma is more common in the geriatric mouse, and different mouse strains have different incidences of neoplasia. Probably all mammary tumors in mice are influenced by the mammary mouse tumor virus transmitted either in germ cells (endogenous form) or in the milk and saliva (exogenous form). The endogenous virus can be incorporated in the mouse genome and be passed in a mendelian fashion.[31] Hormones, stress, and chemical carcinogens also may influence in the development of these tumors. The neoplasms can involve 1 or more glands along the chain, which extends from the axillary to inguinal region. The exogenous form also can cause lymphoma.

Mammary neoplasia commonly infiltrates surrounding tissues.

Spontaneous mammary tumors metastasize with high frequency, but this property is somewhat mouse strain dependent. Metastases primarily go to the lung.

Mammary tumors vary in the types of cell receptors they contain. Ovary-dependent tumors contain estrogen and progesterone receptors, whereas pregnancy-dependent tumors have prolactin receptors. Ovariectomy dramatically reduces the incidence of mammary tumors in certain genetic strains (such as C3H) of mice. If surgery is done in adult mice 2 months to 5 months of age, mammary tumors will develop, but at a later age than normal.

Several other diseases can present in the older mouse. Depending on the organs affected, clinical signs may be noted[32]:

1. Alveolar and/or bronchial epithelium hyperplasia, which can be confused with pulmonary tumors on radiographs. Hyperplasia may be a coincidental finding and no signs are manifested by the pet.
2. Age-associated liver lesions are common and can include biliary hyperplasia, hepatitis, amyloid deposition, fibrosis, hepatomas, and carcinomas. In many cases, therapy is palliative in nature only. The use of liver protectants may benefit mice. One study reported that a silymarin dose of 500 mg/kg, every 24 hours, decreased fatty liver–associated damage.[33]
3. Nearly all strains of mice develop some form of osteoarthrosis. The use of NSAIDs is indicated.
4. Kidney lesions, such as glomerulonephritis. It is associated more often with persistent viral infections or immune disorders rather than with bacterial infections. Signs include muscle wasting, weight loss, and proteinuria. It is progressive. Force-feeding a liquid gruel and/or subcutaneous fluids may prolong quality of life.

Hamsters

Hamsters as pets include the Syrian (also called teddy bear) hamster, Campbell dwarf hamster, Roborovski dwarf hamster, Russian winter white hamster, and Chinese hamster. The life span typically is no more than 2 years.

Diseases affecting the geriatric hamster include dilated cardiomyopathy, atrial thrombosis, amyloidosis of various organs, hyperadrenocorticism, and neoplasia.[10,34,35]

Dilated cardiomyopathy and atrial thrombosis have common nonspecific signs, such as lethargy, anorexia, and tachypnea. There is a correlation with atrial thrombosis. Radiography and ultrasonography may aid in the diagnosis. Therapy is symptomatic and can include diuretics and other cardiac medications, as shown in above table.

The incidence of atrial thrombosis is influenced by the endocrine status of the animal, especially by the amount of circulating androgens. As a result, castration of male Syrian hamsters is linked to an increase in the prevalence of atrial thrombosis.[36] Disseminated intravascular coagulation has been found in conjunction with cases of atrial thrombosis.

Amyloidosis is common in the geriatric hamster and may be a coincidental finding. Amyloid is an insoluble pathologic proteinaceous substance, deposited between cells in various tissues and organs of the body. Amyloid deposits are more common in female hamsters greater than 1.5 years of age. Deposits can be seen in the liver, kidney, spleen, and adrenal glands as well as occasionally in almost any other organ. Diagnosis is made on histopathology. Signs depend on the organ affected. Depending on the organ affected, therapy is directed at supporting that organ function (such as subcutaneous fluids if the kidneys are affected).

Neoplasia can affect a variety of organs. Treatment usually is palliative, with some neoplasia amenable to surgery.

Approximately 30% of Syrian hamsters have neoplasms, with no appreciable sex difference in the overall tumor incidence. The most frequent tumor types were those of the adrenal cortex (13.5%), the lymphoreticular system (3%), and the endometrium (3%). Small intestinal adenocarcinomas occurred in 0.8% of the animals.[37]

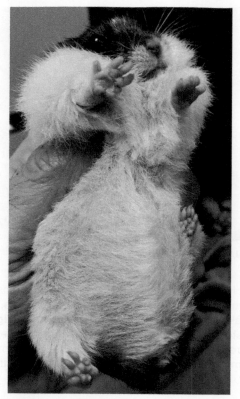

Fig. 23. Thinning fur on gerbil with hyperadrenocorticism.

In older Syrian hamsters, lymphoma is the most frequently observed neoplasm of the hematopoietic system. It is multicentric and commonly affects lymphatic organs.[36] It is speculated that some of these adult-onset lymphomas may be transmissible tumors that capitalize on the homozygosity of Syrian hamsters.

Cutaneous lymphoma (or epitheliotropic lymphoma) also can occur. Diagnosis is made based on histopathology. Depending on the location, some may be removed surgically.

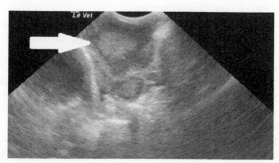

Fig. 24. Ultrasound of same gerbil with adrenal gland enlargement (*white arrow*) confirmed by histopathology.

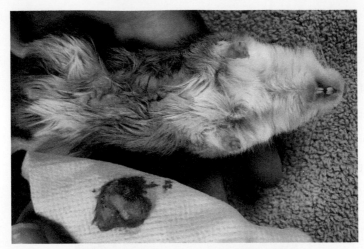

Fig. 25. Histopathology confirmed scent gland carcinoma in a gerbil.

Hyperadrenocorticism occurs commonly, usually in male hamsters, and is associated with bilateral symmetric alopecia of flanks and lateral thighs, thinning and hyperpigmentation of the skin, polydipsia, polyuria, and polyphagia (**Fig. 23**). Research has suggested that hamsters may secrete both cortisol and corticosterone, making confirmation with dynamic assays difficult.[38] Enlarged adrenal glands may be located on ultrasonography in some cases (**Fig. 24**). A consistent successful therapy has not been reported to date.

Gerbils

Gerbils live 2 years to 5 years, with the occasional reported pet living to 8 years of age.

Commonly reported diseases of geriatric gerbils include scent gland neoplasms, cystic ovaries, chronic interstitial nephritis, and cerebral vascular ischemia (stroke).

Ventral marking, gland hyperplasia, and carcinomas (**Fig. 25**) are common in older gerbils (>1.5 years). They present as small, possible reddish, waxy skin masses over the umbilicus. Diagnosis is made by histopathology and treatment is surgical removal. If neoplastic, they may recur.

Cystic ovaries are common in gerbils over 1 year of age and clinical signs include symmetric alopecia, abdominal swelling, lethargy, anorexia, dyspnea, and reduced fertility. Diagnosis can be made on physical examination and ultrasonography. Therapy is an ovariectomy or ovariohysterectomy.

Chronic interstitial nephritis is a common finding. If the gerbil is clinical for this disease, signs include polyuria, proteinuria, lethargy, and proteinuria. Treatment is supportive in nature.

In mammals, the circle of Willis is composed of a communication of arteries at the bottom of the brain, consisting of the internal carotid arteries, anterior cerebral arteries, anterior communicating arteries, posterior communicating arteries, posterior cerebral arteries, and basilar arteries. This structure provides for alternate blood flow to the brain in case 1 artery becomes occluded.

Some gerbils do not have an anatomically complete circle of Willis and may be prone to cerebral ischemia. Gerbils are used as a human model for cerebral ischemia, and research has shown several pharmaceuticals may help in protecting neuronal tissue, especially in the acute phase. From a clinical perspective, most of these pharmaceuticals are not commonly found in the veterinary pharmacy. Steroids do not appear to be beneficial in return to function.[39]

Cerebral ischemia signs include paralysis, inability to open 1 or both eyes, head tilt, and/or incoordination. Therapy includes supportive treatment of subcutaneous fluids, force-feeding, and maintenance of normal body temperature. Anecdotally, gerbils may benefit from NSAIDs. Many gerbils recover with a residual head tilt.

DISCLOSURE

The authors have nothing to disclose.

REFERENCES

1. Johnson-Delaney CA. Geriatric Care of Rabbits and Rodents. Wild West Veterinary Conference 2011.
2. Taylor BF, Ramirez HE, Battles AH, et al. Analgesic activity of tramadol and buprenorphine after voluntary ingestion by rats (Rattus norvegicus). J Am Assoc Lab Anim Sci 2016;55(1):74–82.
3. Wodarrski R, Clark AK, Grist J, et al. Gabapentin reverses microglial activation in the spinal cord of streptozotocin-induced diabetic rats. Eur J Pain 2009;13(8): 807–11.
4. Vollmer KO, von Hodenberg A, Kölle EU. Pharmacokinetics and metabolism of gabapentin in rat, dog and man. Arzneimittelforschung 1986;36(5):830–9.
5. Gauchan P, Andoh T, Ikeda K, et al. Mechanical allodynia induced by paclitaxel, oxaliplatin and vincristine: different effectiveness of gabapentin and different expression of voltage-dependent calcium channel alpha(2)delta-1 subunit. Biol Pharm Bull 2009;32(4):732–4.
6. Ewing LE, Skinner CM, Quick CM, et al. Hepatotoxicity of a cannabidiol-rich cannabis extract in the mouse model. Molecules 2019;24(9) [pii:E1694].
7. Hammell DC, Zhang LP, Ma F, et al. Transdermal cannabidiol reduces inflammation and pain-related behaviours in a rat model of arthritis. Eur J Pain 2016;20(6): 936–48.
8. Braida D, Pegorini S, Arcidiacono MV, et al. Post-ischemic treatment with cannabidiol prevents electroencephalographic flattening, hyperlocomotion and neuronal injury in gerbils. Neurosci Lett 2003;346(1–2):61–4.
9. Quesenberry K, Carpenter J. Ferrets, rabbits, and rodents. Clinical medicine and surgery. 3rd edition 2011.
10. Heatley JJ. Cardiovascular anatomy, physiology, and disease of rodents and small exotic mammals. Vet Clin Exot Anim Pract 2009;12(1):99–113.
11. BSAVA Small Animal Formulary 7th edition.
12. Jin H, Nishino T, Aoe T, et al. A simple and safe method for tracheal intubation using a supraglottic intubation-aid device in mice. Respir Physiol Neurobiol 2019;263:9–13.
13. Cheong SH, Lee JH, Kim MH, et al. Airway management using a supraglottic airway device without endotracheal intubation for positive ventilation of anaesthetized rats. Lab Anim 2013;47:89–93.
14. Tamura Y. Current approach to rodents as patients. J Exot Pet Med 2010;19(1): 36–55. Standards of Care.
15. Coutant T, Vergneau-Grosset C, Langlois I. Overview of drug delivery methods in exotics, including their anatomic and physiologic considerations. Vet Clin Exot Anim Pract 2018;21(2):215–59.
16. VIN Formulary for Exotic Animals.

17. BSAVA Small Animal Formulary 8th edition.
18. Hocker SE, Eshar D, Wouda RM. Rodent oncology. Vet Clin Exot Anim Pract 2017; 20(1):111–34.
19. Hotchkiss CE. Effect of surgical removal of subcutaneous tumors on survival of rats. J Am Vet Med Assoc 1995;206:1575–9.
20. Dragan YP, Fahey S, Street K, et al. Studies of tamoxifen as a promoter of hepatocarcinogenesis in female Fischer F344 rats. Breast Cancer Res Treat 1994;31:11–25.
21. Keenan K, Smith PF, Hertzog P, et al. The effects of overfeeding and dietary restriction on Sprague-Dawley rat survival and early pathology biomarkers of aging. Toxicol Pathol 1994;22(3):300–15.
22. Mayer J, Sato A, Kiupel M, et al. Extralabel use of cabergoline in the treatment of a pituitary adenoma in a rat. J Am Vet Med Assoc 2011;239:656–60.
23. Tucker MJ. The effect of long-term food restriction on tumours in rodents. Int J Cancer 1979;23:803–7.
24. Percy DH, Barthold SW. Rat. In: Pathology of laboratory rodents & rabbits. 2nd edition. Ames (IA): Iowa State University Press; 2001. p. 107–58.
25. Donnelly T. Disease problems of small rodents. In: Quesenberry KE, Carpenter JW, editors. Ferrets, rabbits and rodents: clinical medicine and surgery. 2nd edition. Philadelphia: WB Saunders; 2004. p. 305–8.
26. Anver MR, Cohen BJ. Lesions associated with aging. In: Baker HJ, Lindsey JR, Weisbroth SH, editors. The laboratory rat, vol. 1, 1st edition. New York: Academic Press; 1979. p. 378–99.
27. Haines V. The ancient rat. Vet Clin North Am Exot Anim Pract 2010;13(1):15–25.
28. Krinke GJ. Spontaneous radioneuropathology, aged rats. In: Jones TC, Mohr U, Hunt RD, editors. Monographs on pathology of laboratory animals: nervous system. New York: SpringerVerlag; 1988. p. 203–8.
29. Jolivalt CG, Mizisin LM, Nelson A, et al. B vitamins alleviate indices of neuropathic pain in diabetic rats. Eur J Pharmacol 2009;10(612):41–7.
30. Sun H, Yang T, Li Q, et al. Dexamethasone and vitamin B12 synergistically promote peripheral nerve regeneration in rats by upregulating the expression of brain-derived neurotrophic factor. Arch Med Sci 2012;8(5):924–30.
31. MacLachlan NJ, Dubovi EJ, editors. Retroviridae. Fenner's veterinary virology. 5th edition. Elsevier; 2016.
32. Whary MT, Anderson L, Otto G, et al. Biology and diseases of mice. Lab animal medicine. The laboratory rabbit, Guinea pig, Hamster, and other rodents. American College of Laboratory Animal Medicine; 2012.
33. Pais P, D'Amato M. In vivo efficacy study of milk thistle extract (ETHIS-094™) in STAM™ model of nonalcoholic steatohepatitis. Drugs R D 2014;14(4):291–9.
34. Karolewski B, Mayer TW, Ruble G. Non-infectious diseases. Lab animal medicine. The laboratory rabbit, Guinea pig, Hamster, and other rodents. American College of Laboratory Animal Medicine; 2012.
35. Schmidt RE, Reavill DR. Cardiovascular disease in hamsters: review and retrospective study. J Exot Pet Med 2007;16(1):49–51.
36. Merck Veterinary Manual. Accessed October 18, 2019.
37. Fabry A. The incidence of neoplasms in Syrian hamsters with particular emphasis on intestinal neoplasia. Arch Toxicol Suppl 1985;8:124–7.
38. Brown C, Donnelly TM. Disease problems of small rodents. In: Quesenberry K, Ferrets CJ, editors. Rabbits, and rodents. Clinical medicine and surgery. 3rd edition; 2011.
39. McGraw CP, Fleming DF, Spruil JH. Effect of methylprednisolone on experimental cerebral infarction in the Mongolian Gerbil. Stroke 1974;5:444–5.

Geriatric Ferrets

Cathy A. Johnson-Delaney, DVM*

KEYWORDS

- Geriatric ferret • Neoplasia • Cardiomyopathy • Dental disease • Renal disease

KEY POINTS

- Ferrets become geriatric at 3 years of age.
- The geriatric ferret work-up should include a physical examination, dental examination, bloodwork, and imaging.
- Neoplastic diseases effect nearly all geriatric ferrets and include adrenal, insulinoma, lymphoma, and skin tumors.
- Cardiomyopathy, dental disease, chronic gastrointestinal disorders, and renal disease are commonly found in geriatric ferrets.
- Musculoskeletal disorders include spondylosis, spondylitis, and arthritis.

INTRODUCTION

Pet ferrets live an average of 5 to 7 years. They are considered geriatric at 3 years of age. This young age in the owner's eyes may make it difficult for them to accept that their ferret needs additional veterinary care. The veterinarian needs to develop a health care plan for the aging ferret, and discuss the importance of maintaining a good quality of life for the pet. Discussing aging and death with owners who are deeply bonded to their ferret, particularly if the family includes children, is difficult. Having a program in place that provides information about end-of-life scenarios can serve to educate the owner about clinical signs they may see in their aging ferret. Ferrets may hide symptoms of pain and distress, holding off showing overt illness as long as possible. Close observations of demeanor, posture, alertness, eye character, appetite, drinking, urination, defecation (including stool consistency), activity, and responses to other ferrets, pets, and the owners are used to determine if a ferret is experiencing pain or distress. Geriatric ferrets have a high likelihood of one or more neoplasias. They also commonly have cardiac, dental, gastrointestinal, and renal diseases. Splenomegaly is a common finding and is often caused by extramedullary hematopoiesis rather than a neoplastic process. Cataracts are fairly common and must be differentiated from lenticular sclerosis. Musculoskeletal conditions include osteoarthritis, spondylosis, and disc disease. Geriatric ferrets may require extensive medical and surgical treatments to

Special Projects, NW Zoological Supply, Everett, WA, USA
* 13818 65th Avenue West, #7, Edmonds, WA 98026.
E-mail address: cajddvm@hotmail.com

Vet Clin Exot Anim 23 (2020) 549–565
https://doi.org/10.1016/j.cvex.2020.04.002
1094-9194/20/© 2020 Elsevier Inc. All rights reserved.

vetexotic.theclinics.com

maintain a good quality of life. Complementary therapies, such as nutraceuticals, herbals, acupuncture, and therapeutic lasers, may also contribute to keeping the ferret comfortable.

VETERINARY ASSESSMENT

A geriatric ferret ideally should have a physical examination twice yearly. A detailed history of diet and appetite and the owner's observations of bowel and urinary action should be taken. Activity levels, play duration, and behaviors should be discussed. The examination should include an ophthalmic examination to differentiate between lenticular sclerosis and cataracts. Tonometry should be done to rule out glaucoma. Otoscopic examination is done to check the integrity of the tympanic membrane and the condition of the ear canal and pinna. It may be necessary to remove wax build-up before the otoscope cone insertion. Wax removed should be microscopically examined for the presence of *Otodectes cynotis*. Dental and oral examination should be done, with dental radiographs planned if any abnormalities are seen. Otherwise dental radiographs may be taken annually. Dental prophylaxis under anesthesia is recommended annually. The ferret is palpated easily and any organomegaly, masses, or areas of pain can be found. Cardiac examination should include auscultation with Doppler audio of the heart valves. Palpation of the chest is done to assess compressibility of the thorax and the size of the heart. If cardiomegaly is present and/or if arrythmia is detected, electrocardiography and echocardiography should be done. Blood pressure determination is done, although it is a challenge in an awake ferret because of the size of even the smallest cuff: determinations are most commonly done on the front leg or tail base. The examination should include hematology and serum chemistries and urinalysis including refractometry for specific gravity. The chemistry panel should include a fasting blood glucose. Fasting duration for a ferret is 2 to 4 hours. If the ferret has a history of insulinoma or suspected hypoglycemic episodes, 2 hours is sufficient. Insulin level taken at the time of a low fasting blood glucose level is useful in determining the presence of insulinoma. Additional blood testing may be warranted if endocrine disorders are suspected (eg, sex steroids and thyroid parameters). Whole-body radiographs and thoracic and abdominal ultrasonography should be done at least annually or more frequently if abnormalities are found. Additional examinations including biopsies, computed tomography (CT) scans, or other laboratory testing should be initiated based on physical findings. Vaccinations given should follow risk assessment or regulatory requirements. Rabies vaccination annually is mandated in some states or municipal jurisdictions. Canine distemper virus titer level is useful to determine how frequently canine distemper virus vaccination is needed rather than just annually as per the manufacturer. Although ferrets are susceptible to human influenza, and the commercial human influenza vaccines are effective in ferrets, routine vaccination for influenza is not usually done. It is recommended that owners and humans in contact with ferrets be vaccinated annually for influenza to protect the ferret. Many ferrets are now on a program to prevent clinical adrenal disease and have been implanted with 4.7 mg deslorelin acetate (Suprelorin-F, Virbac, Ft. Worth, TX) starting usually in their first year, although some ferrets have not received implants until they have been diagnosed with adrenal disease. For most ferrets, it is being recommended that they receive a repeat implant every 12 to 16 months. The implantation schedule should be tailored to the individual ferret and incorporated into their life health plan. Suggested guidelines for geriatric ferret health management are in **Table 1**.[1]

Table 1	
Suggested geriatric ferret screening	
Between 3 and 6 y of age	Examination including physical, radiographs every 6 mo
	Bloodwork (CBC, chemistries including fasting glucose [2 h], urinalysis) every 6–12 mo
	Dental prophylaxis at least annually; dental radiographs at least annually
	Ophthalmic, otoscopic examination annually
	Cardiac evaluation at least annually; in endemic areas, heartworm ELISA-antigen testing and prophylaxis
	Ultrasonography: abdominal, echocardiograph at least annually
	Vaccinations: risk assessment, serology, administration if indicated
	Additional endocrine, imaging, diagnostic testing as indicated
Older than 6 y of age: every 6 mo	Examination including physical, radiology, ultrasonography
	Cardiac evaluation; in endemic areas, heartworm ELISA-antigen testing and prophylaxis
	Ophthalmic, otoscopic examination
	Bloodwork, urinalysis
	Dental radiographs and prophylaxis
	Additional endocrine, imaging, diagnostic testing as indicated
	Vaccinations for annual administration dependent on risk assessment

Abbreviations: CBC, complete blood count; ELISA, enzyme-linked immunosorbent assay.

DIETARY CONSIDERATIONS

At present, studies have not been done evaluating lowered protein levels in aging ferrets, particularly those with elevated blood urea nitrogen and/or creatinine levels, as have been done in aging cats and dogs with renal disease. Commercial diets for aging ferrets that have lower protein levels than maintenance diets are available, although benefits have not been evaluated. Most ferrets are maintained on a good quality commercial ferret food for their entire lives and the diet is not changed when they become geriatric. If a ferret has problems masticating dry kibble because of tooth loss, dook soup is fed (**Box 1**).

The geriatric ferret should have food and water bowls that are easily accessible. The sipper tube of a water bottle should be positioned so that the ferret can comfortably drink. If the ferret is having problems ambulating, food and water may be provided in multiple locations.

Supplementation with omega 3-6-9 fatty acids may have benefits based on evidence in other species. Geriatric ferrets may also benefit from additional supplements, such as L-carnitine and taurine for the heart and muscles, coenzyme Q_{10} to support metabolism, milk thistle (silybins) to support the liver, vitamin E and hawthorn to support the heart, and chondroitin sulfate/glucosamine to support joint health. Usage of supplements and their benefits in ferrets is anecdotal. **Box 2** is an example of a supplement formula for use in geriatric ferrets.

HUSBANDRY CONSIDERATIONS

As a ferret ages, climbing multiple levels and having to climb into a hammock may be difficult. A ferret with weakness or musculoskeletal problems may slip and fall in a

Box 1
Dook soup: recipe for approximately one meal

Ingredients
  Pulverized or ground kibble (what the ferret is normally used to eating), powder consistency.
  Measuring spoons, mixing bowl, spoons, 30-mL syringe/feeding syringe.
  Water or organic low-sodium chicken broth.
  Chicken or turkey baby food, or cooked chicken puree (thoroughly cook a chicken including bones, process so that the bones are ground into it; puree. Portions of this can be frozen in ice cube trays, then one cube is used for each meal).
  Carnivore Care (Oxbow Pet Products, Omaha, NE) or Emeraid Carnivore (Emeraid LLC, Cornell, IL).
  Nutri-cal gel (Vetoquinol, Ft. Worth, TX).

Procedure
  Mix 1 teaspoon kibble powder with enough water or broth to make it fluid. It may need to soak for more than an hour.
  Add in 1 heaping teaspoon of Carnivore Care plus enough water or broth to make it soup.
  For extra calories and to increase palatability, add in 0.5–1 teaspoon of Nutri-cal (optional).
  Mix in 1 heaping teaspoon of baby food/chicken puree.
  Stir well. Additional water/broth may be needed to adjust consistency.

Feed to the ferret: off a spoon, finger, or using a feeding syringe. A meal is usually 30 mL of this soup per 1-kg ferret at least 3 times a day. Volume or frequency are altered to prevent weight loss. If the ferret eats the soup on its own out of a bowl, a continued supply is provided for ad lib feeding.

Box 2
Geriatric ferret formula

Ingredients
  1000 mg L-carnitine
  1000 mg taurine
  1000 mg coenzyme Q_{10}
  400 IU vitamin E
  80–100 mg hawthorn
  500 mg milk thistle
  1800 mg chondroitin sulfate, 600 mg glucosamine, 16 mg manganese (1 scoop equine Cosequin [Nutramax Labs, Edgewood, MD])
  Omega 3-6-9 oil (VetOmega, Avian Studios, North Salt Lake, UT)
  Small funnel
  2-oz plastic Yorker bottle, marked at the 1-oz level
  Chopstick for stirring
  16–18 gauge needle
  Oral syringe (eg, a 3-mL syringe without needle) for administration

Process
  Using a small funnel in the top of the Yorker bottle, empty capsule contents into the bottle. Pour in 1 scoop of the Cosequin. Remove the funnel. Puncture the coenzyme Q_{10} capsule and express contents into the bottle. Puncture the vitamin E capsule and express contents into the bottle. Pour in a small amount of VetOmega oil and stir with the chopstick. Pour in additional VetOmega to bring the volume up to the 1-oz mark. Stir again.
  Store in the refrigerator.

To use: stir well before measuring out 0.5–1 mL/ferret/24-h period.

multilevel cage. It may be necessary to change the caging to a single level type. Food, water, and sleeping bedding should be easily accessible. The litter box tray rim may need to be lowered for ease of getting into it. Toilet habits may deteriorate so placing the box on papers within the cage may make cleaning up easier. The litter box should be cleaned preferably twice daily.[2]

GENERAL CHANGES IN GERIATRIC FERRETS

Ferrets continue to play throughout life, but an older ferret plays for less time. A ferret that drops to the ground lying flat (called flat-ferret, pelting, or speedbump) after just a few steps needs to be evaluated because this is not a normal symptom of aging. It is more commonly associated with generalized weakness, cardiac insufficiency, hypoglycemia, or musculoskeletal disorders and/or pain. Many aging ferrets get more white or gray hairs throughout their coats, which may give them more of a roan coat. Alopecia is associated with endocrine disease rather than as a function of aging.

SPECIFIC COMMON DISEASES OF GERIATRIC FERRETS
Cardiac Disease

Both dilated (DCM) and hypertrophic (HCM) cardiomyopathy and what is characterized as "mixed" cardiomyopathy (containing elements of dilated and hypertrophic) have been found in geriatric ferrets. Arrhythmias and valvular disease have been documented. Heartworm disease is found in some geographic areas.[2] DCM is the most common, although the exact cause is unknown. It is important to distinguish among the different types of cardiomyopathies before initiating treatment. Cardiac disease is often not detected early in the disease process unless clinicians incorporate screening into examinations starting at 3 years of age. The typical decreased activity associated with cardiac disease is often just interpreted by owners as normal slowing down seen with aging. Cardiomegaly is not diagnostic for the type of cardiac disease (**Fig. 1**).

DCM is found in ferrets older than 3 years of age, with no sex predilection. Although in other species it is linked with taurine deficiency, this link has not been determined in ferrets. Clinical signs are nonspecific for heart disease: exercise intolerance and/or lethargy; weight loss (muscle mass); anorexia; and in some, coughing, distended abdomen, and dyspnea (caused by pulmonary edema). The distended abdomen may be caused by hepatomegaly, splenomegaly, and/or ascites (**Fig. 2**). After auscultation, radiographs followed by echocardiography are indicated. Radiographs should include the thorax and the abdomen. Changes in the thorax may include an elevated trachea or increased sternal contact with the heart, and/or cardiomegaly including a globoid appearance or the appearance of bulging atria. Echocardiography differentiates among DCM, HCM, mixed cardiomyopathy, pericardial effusion, and thoracic masses, and eliminates adult heartworm presence from the differentials.[3] Testing for the presence of heartworms in endemic areas should also include enzyme-linked immunosorbent assay–based antigen tests, although because of low worm burdens, false-negative test results occur. Treatment includes ultrasound-guided retrieval of heartworms and/or ivermectin, cage rest, and steroids to reduce inflammation.[4]

Mitral valve murmurs are not uncommon in ferrets and may be associated with DCM or valvular disease. If auscultated, the murmur should be pursued with further diagnostics, such as audio Doppler and echocardiography. Arrhythmias found on general auscultation should also be pursued with electrocardiography. These can include tachycardia, bradycardia, premature ventricular complexes, or other abnormalities.

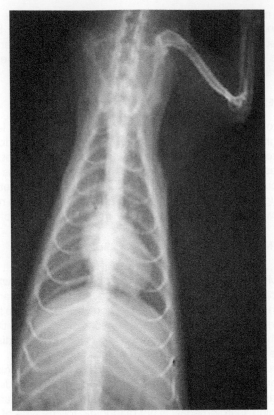

Fig. 1. Cardiomegaly on ventrodorsal radiograph. Further diagnostics are needed to determine the contributing cardiomyopathy. Vertebral heart score (VHS) in ferrets may indicate cardiomegaly, but should only be part of a full cardiac workup. The normal ferret VHS for the lateral view is 3.75 to 4.07 vertebrae.

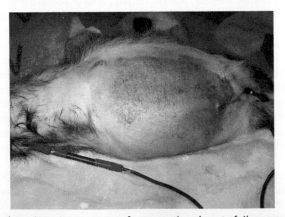

Fig. 2. Abdominal ascites in a case of congestive heart failure caused by dilated cardiomyopathy.

Many arrhythmias respond to medical treatment and correcting any other underlying medical conditions including electrolyte imbalances, although pacemaker implantation has been done in ferrets.[1,2]

Treatments are similar to those used in dogs and cats for the definitive cardiomyopathy. Initially oxygen therapy is used for ferrets with dyspnea. Furosemide is used to decrease pulmonary edema at 2 to 2.5 mg/kg every 8 to 12 hours. For DCM, initial therapy may be with digoxin at 0.01 mg/kg every 24 hours for the first few days; however, using a phosphodiesterase inhibitor that increases cardiac contractility, such as pimobendan, has less chance of causing toxicity and can be used as the maintenance medication. It is also used in valvular disease. Dosage starts at 0.5 mg/kg orally every 12 hours. Angiotensin-converting enzyme inhibitors, such as enalapril at 0.25 to 0.5 mg/kg every 24 to 48 hours, may also be used for some ferrets early in the disease process, or adjunctively with pimobendan. HCM therapy usually includes β-blockers, such as atenolol at 3 to 6 mg/kg orally every 24 hours or a calcium channel blocker, such as diltiazem at 1.5 to 7.5 mg/kg orally every 12 hours. The author also places ferrets with any type of heart disease on a supplement (Geriatric Ferret Formula, **Box 2**).[1,2,5]

Ferrets can have heart attacks with resultant ischemic infarctions. The myocardial damage may not be found until necropsy. A ferret that presents experiencing such an episode may be semiconscious, tachypneic, with cold extremities. Cardiac rhythm may be erratic and/or bradycardic: attachment to an electrocardiogram should be part of the emergency procedure. Oxygen should be provided. Intravenous dobutamine, atropine, and lidocaine is used to stabilize the heart. The intraosseous route is used if a vein cannot quickly be accessed. The author has successfully managed many ferrets presented during a cardiac event. Having an emergency kit for ferrets that includes these drugs and ferret dosages readily available is easily assembled. Emergency conditions in ferrets and their treatments are beyond the scope of this article.

Dental Disease

Geriatric ferrets present with calculi, gingivitis, periodontitis, fractured teeth, worn teeth, and even dental abscesses (tooth root abscesses, usually following fractured teeth with open pulp cavities) (**Fig. 3**).[1,2] It is fairly common to see the tips of the canine

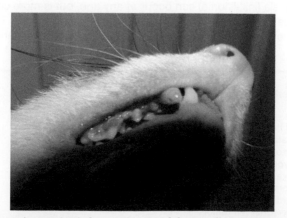

Fig. 3. Dental disease in a geriatric ferret. The tip of the maxillary canine tooth is broken off. There is calculi and mild gingivitis.

teeth broken off, which may or may not have exposed the pulp cavity. Gum recession especially around the base of the canines can be pronounced in older ferrets. Clinical signs of dental disease may include anorexia, bruxism, halitosis, and hypersalivation. A thorough dental examination should include dental radiographs, and periodontal probing and measurements. Extractions of necrotic teeth may be curative. Although root canal of canine teeth is possible, because of their small size and curvature, it is difficult. Regular prophylaxis under anesthesia is performed as in dogs and cats. Owners should be encouraged to brush their ferret's teeth routinely. An enzymatic toothpaste as used in dogs and cats works well in ferrets.[1]

Endocrine Diseases

Endocrinopathies receive the most attention in aging ferrets, although they also can begin in young ferrets.[6] Adrenal disease and islet cell neoplasia (insulinoma) are the most common, but diabetes mellitus, pheochromocytomas, hypothyroidism, hypoparathyroidism, hypoadrenocorticism, and varying degrees of malignancies have been documented.[6–12] Many ferrets have more than one endocrinopathy.[13,14] A full discussion of endocrine disease is beyond the scope of this article. A list of endocrine neoplasias is shown in **Box 3**.[6]

Adrenal disease is characterized by elevations in one or more of the sex steroids, even in neutered ferrets. The hormone elevations and accompanying clinical signs can occur with all stages of the disease: hyperplasia, adenoma, and adenocarcinoma. Clinical signs include behavioral changes (aggression), pruritis, enlarged vulva, enlarged prostate (including cysts), alopecia, comedones, thinning of the skin, and even weight loss.[15] Diagnosis starts with hematology, serum biochemistries, radiographs, and abdominal ultrasound; in males, this should include the prostate. Serum sex hormone levels are useful to assess level of the disease and are repeated to monitor treatment. Although adrenalectomy may be necessary if there is organ displacement, depending on the age of the ferret and other disease conditions (eg, cardiomyopathy) therapy usually starts with sex steroid suppression using a gonadotropin-releasing hormone agonist, such as leuprolide acetate depot formulation or deslorelin.[16,17] If the prostate is involved, additional antiandrogen medications, such as finasteride or bicalutamide, help provide immediate local sex steroid receptor blocking. Prostatic cysts are aspirated using ultrasound guidance. Maintaining urinary patency is a priority in male ferrets with adrenal disease.

Islet cell neoplasia (insulinoma) can occur at any age, but is more common in older ferrets. β-Cell adenoma and adenocarcinomas have been reported. The tumors may be in visible discrete nodules or microscopic and diffuse within the pancreas. They are

---

Box 3
Endocrine neoplasias

Tumor type
  Adrenocortical neoplasms
  Islet cell neoplasia (insulinoma)
  Pheochromocytoma
  Pancreatic polypeptidoma
  Thyroid adenocarcinoma
  Pituitary adenoma
  Ovarian sex-cord stromal tumors
  Sertoli cell, interstitial cell tumors
  C-cell carcinoma

functional and secrete insulin, with clinical signs linked to hypoglycemia and include collapse, seizures, retching, hypersalivation, tearing at the mouth, and nausea. The tumors can metastasize most commonly into the liver. Diagnosis is with repeated blood glucose levels and paired with insulin levels. Imaging, such as CT or ultrasound, may show nodules.[18] Treatment usually begins medically managing the hypoglycemia with frequent meals, prednisolone, and diazoxide. Surgical removal of nodules or portions of the pancreas is done as well. Even with surgery, there is usually recurrence.

Gastrointestinal Diseases

Inflammatory bowel disease or irritable bowel disease, ulcerative colitis, lymphoma, hepatitis/hepatopathy, biliary disorders including gallstones, and trichobezoars have all been associated with aging in ferrets.[1,2] Gastric and/or duodenal ulcers may be linked to chronic administration of medications, such as prednisone, or form associated with the stresses from any disease process. Diarrhea and anorexia are the most common presenting signs of gastrointestinal disease. Pain or discomfort on abdominal palpation may be present along with organomegaly, enlarged mesenteric lymph nodes, gas/fluid presence in bowel loops, and changes in borborygmus on abdominal auscultation. Diagnostics include bloodwork, radiographs (possibly with contrast study), abdominal ultrasonography, fecal examination (flotation, smear, cytology, Gram stain, possibly culture), and in some cases laparotomy with biopsies.

Inflammatory bowel disease is a chronic condition, and like in other species, seems to be multifactorial and progressive.[19] Ferrets will have diarrhea, that varies in character and may be intermittent. Slow loss of body condition and weight loss are part of the clinical picture. Definitive diagnosis is with full-thickness gastric and intestinal biopsies, which differentiate between inflammatory bowel disease (eosinophilic, lymphoplasmocytic inflammation) and lymphoma. Treatments may include azathioprine and/or prednisone. Although a hypoallergenic diet is always proposed, this may be difficult to do because elimination diets/commercial preparations for ferrets are not available. Feline diets have been used, although efficacy studies have not been done.

Musculoskeletal Disorders

Ferrets can develop spondylosis, spondylitis, and ruptured or compressed discs. Changes in the spinal column may not be clinically apparent unless a ferret falls, and then experiences acute pain, paresis, or paralysis. More subtle and chronic signs of spinal disorders are reluctance to climb or jump; muscle spasms along the spine, particularly in the lumbar area; pain associated with the spine; paresis in the hindquarters; and changes in urination/defecation. Palpation and a detailed neurologic examination, along with radiographs, usually show boney changes. CT and/or MRI are extremely useful in pinpointing lesions. This may be necessary to rule out intraspinal neoplasia, such as lymphoma, which is not uncommon.[20] A myelogram can be performed, although because of the size of the spinal canal, the procedure may be difficult. Prognosis and treatment options depend on diagnosis. Nonsteroidal anti-inflammatory drugs and analgesics should be started immediately. Supportive care may include manual bladder expression, massage, physical therapy, and changing the ferret's housing to prevent climbing and further injury.

Myasthenia gravis has been documented in older ferrets. Clinical signs include anorexia, progressive, generalized muscle weakness, and exercise intolerance. Hematology, serum biochemistries, and radiography may be within normal limits. Diagnosis is made with electromyelography and serologic testing for acetylcholine receptor antibodies.[21] A single dose of neostigmine methylsulfate at 0.04 mg/kg intravenously can be administered. A positive test shows marked lessening of clinical signs for up to 6 hours. Treatment with pyridostigmine and prednisolone may be successful.[21]

Neoplastic Diseases

Although neoplasias in most species are usually associated with advancing age, many are found in young ferrets. The most common ones include adrenocortical adenoma/adenocarcinoma, islet cell neoplasia (insulinoma, discussed previously), and lymphoma (various tissues) with incidence increasing in older ferrets. Many ferrets have multiple tumors of different types all at the same time. Detailed pathology of the many tumors is beyond the scope of this article, but have been well-described.[22] Many types of tumors are documented in geriatric ferrets and are listed in **Table 2** (**Figs. 4** and **5**).

A ferret-specific formula for body surface area has been developed to improve chemotherapeutic dosing.[23] Based on a CT-derived body surface area measurements, the formula is 9.94 + (body weight) (2/3). It is similar to the feline-derived formula most frequently used by practitioners.

Skin tumors are more likely to be found in ferrets older than age 3. These include mast cell tumors, sebaceous epitheliomas, fibromas/fibroadenomas, and many others (**Fig. 6**). Sebaceous epitheliomas and mast cell tumors are benign, and easily surgically removed. Small tumors are treated with cryosurgery; however, surgical removal allows for submission of the mass for histopathology. Unlike mast cell tumors in other species, in ferrets they do not metastasize, although they may occur at other sites after removal at the initial site. They do not carry a poor prognosis even if they keep occurring. Initially owners may opt to treat topically with an over-the-counter antihistamine cream because they can be pruritic and may bleed locally. Preputial tumors are of apocrine gland origin and are malignant with metastasis to surrounding tissues and often into the body wall. Surgical resection should include at least a 1-cm margin, although this may involve partial resection of the penis. There is a report of radiation therapy being tried for these tumors, although results were not always successful.[24]

Ophthalmic Disease

Ferrets experience lenticular sclerosis of the lens as is seen in other animals. They also can develop cataracts.[2] In rare instances the cataracts may lead to a secondary glaucoma. Cataracts may be unilateral or bilateral in formation (**Fig. 8**). Most ferrets retain some degree of light/dark sensation, but are functionally blind. A blind ferret can still navigate well and many owners are not even aware of problem. A full ophthalmic examination including tonometry should be done as part of a geriatric physical examination. Cataracts are removed, although unless one becomes dislocated or there is pain involved (usually glaucoma is present), many owners decide against ophthalmic surgery. An offer to a referral ophthalmologist should be made as part of presenting owners with optimal care for their ferret. Owners should be counseled on ways to make the home safer for a vision-impaired ferret including not altering cage furnishings, dishes, location of litter boxes, major room changes, or allowing the ferret access to stairways.

Renal Disease

Illness associated with renal disease in geriatric ferrets is not well-described, although renal pathology is found in almost all at necropsy.[1,2,36] Signs associated with renal disease tend to be nonspecific and can also be found with many other diseases. These include weakness, exercise intolerance, posterior paresis, lethargy, decreases in appetite, depressed mental attitude, weight loss, muscle mass loss, poor hair coat,

Table 2
Reported nonendocrine neoplasias in geriatric ferrets

Tumor	References
Anal sac adenocarcinoma	25
Astrocytoma	26
Basal cell (sebaceous epithelioma, adenoma)	2,26
Biliary adenoma, adenocarcinoma, cystadenoma	26,27
Bladder carcinoma	26
Ceruminous gland adenocarcinoma	28
Chondrosarcoma	2
Chordoma	2,29
Choroid plexus papilloma	26
Fibroma, fibrosarcoma	1,30
Ganglioneuroma	26
Granular cell tumor	26
Hemangioma, hemangiosarcoma	2
Hepatocellular adenoma, carcinoma	26,27
Lachrymal gland basal cell adenocarcinoma	31
Leiomyoma, leiomyosarcoma	26,27,30
Leukemia	26,27
Lipoma, liposarcoma	26,30
Lymphoma, lymphosarcoma (**Fig. 7**)	1,2,20,26,27,32
Malignant melanoma	33
Malignant mesenchymoma	27
Mammary gland adenoma, adenocarcinoma	26,27
Mast cell	1,2,34
Melanocytoma	30
Meningioma	26
Mesothelioma (peritoneal)	26
Myeloma, myelolipoma	27
Neuroblastoma	35
Neurofibroma, neurilemmoma, neurofibrosarcoma	27
Osteoma, osteosarcoma	1,2,26
Ovarian spindle cell, thecoma, adenocarcinoma	26,27
Pancreatic adenocarcinoma	2,26
Preputial gland adenocarcinoma, apocrine sweat gland tumor	24,26
Prostate adenocarcinoma	27
Renal transitional cell carcinoma, adenoma, carcinoma, nephroblastoma	26,27
Salivary gland carcinoma	30
Schwannoma	30
Squamous cell carcinoma	27
Synovial cell sarcoma	27
Testicular seminoma, leiomyosarcoma, peripheral nerve sheath tumor	26,27

(*continued on next page*)

Table 2 *(continued)*	
Tumor	**References**
Thymoma	2,26
Tracheal adenosquamous carcinoma	27
Uterine leiomyoma, leiomyosarcoma, teratoma, deciduoma, adenocarcinoma	26,27

Data from Refs.[1,2,20,24–35]

nausea/retching/vomiting, and polyuria/polydipsia. Laboratory diagnostics should include complete blood count, biochemistries, and urinalysis with specific gravity. Although blood urea nitrogen may be elevated, creatinine levels are rarely elevated in ferrets even in severe renal disease. A creatinine level of 2 mg/dL is significant.[2] There may be hyperphosphatemia, elevated plasma proteins, and a nonregenerative anemia. Protein electrophoresis should be run to rule out infectious diseases, such as Aleutian disease. The specific gravity shows isosthenuria.[37]

Chronic interstitial nephritis may begin at 2 years of age, and although it is considered progressive, it may not lead to renal failure. Renal cysts are fairly common and can become large. They are often incidental findings, and are usually not associated with renal disease. They are distinguished from hydronephrosis with ultrasonography and excretory urograms. Hydronephrosis can compromise kidney function, and may occur in older ferrets with urinary obstruction (prostatic enlargement, urolithiasis, neoplasia). If the obstruction is alleviated before renal failure, then the ferret may clinically have no further renal impairment. Older ferrets may develop glomerulosclerosis and renal hypertension. Twice-yearly serum chemistries including electrolytes along with monitoring peripheral blood pressure and cardiac function can manage these age-related conditions. This includes antihypertensive medications and correction of electrolyte imbalances.

Although commercial lower protein diets are sold for geriatric ferrets, there is a paucity of data to show that decreasing the dietary protein has any effect on renal function. In the author's opinion, it is more important to keep the ferret eating a good-quality ferret diet as it ages than to decrease protein based on extrapolations from cats. Ferret nutritional requirements, anatomy, and physiology vary significantly from cats.

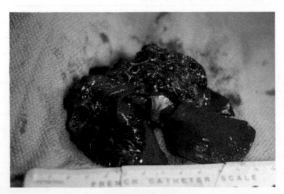

Fig. 4. Hepatocellular carcinoma in a geriatric ferret.

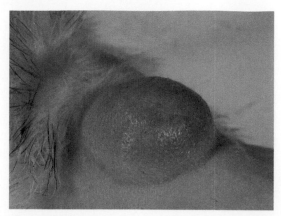

Fig. 5. Lipoma in a 6-year-old ferret.

Splenomegaly

Most older ferrets develop some degree of splenomegaly.[1] The most common cause is extramedullary hematopoiesis as the spleen assumes red cell production in addition to production in bone marrow or in many cases because of decreased bone marrow production.[2] It is found when other medical conditions increase the demand for tissue oxygen, such as with cardiomyopathy. The spleen may be many times normal size, but is smooth in texture and usually homogenous on ultrasonography. Lymphoma, cysts, and hemangioma/hemangiosarcoma can be involved with splenomegaly and splenectomy may be necessary. Splenic biopsies are performed by ultrasound-guided biopsy needles or during abdominal surgery. Unless the spleen is compromising the ferret's ability to ambulate, or there is definitive pathology, the spleen is not removed. A spleen should not be removed without first doing a bone marrow biopsy to assess red blood cell production.

Miscellaneous Conditions Reported in Geriatric Ferrets

Chylous ascites has been reported in 2- to 7-year-old ferrets. One was caused by an obstruction of lymphatic drainage from lymphoma and the second case developed as a postoperative complication from metastatic adrenal carcinoma.[38]

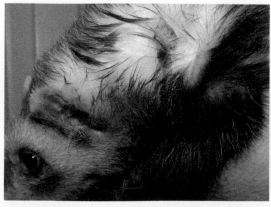

Fig. 6. Mast cell tumor on a 5-year-old ferret.

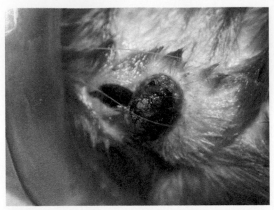

Fig. 7. Lymphoma at the lateral canthi in a geriatric ferret.

Mesenteric heterotopic ossificans was diagnosed in a 5-year-old ferret. The soft tissue ossification involved the omentum. The cause was unknown.[39]

QUALITY OF LIFE

Ferrets may hide signs of serious illness, which has led erroneously to the idea that they are "stoic." This makes determining a plan for hospice care and the end of life a difficult one for owners and the veterinarian. A plan enables the owner to evaluate the quality of life of the ferret, work with the family to deal with the upcoming loss, and alleviate feelings of guilt. The owner needs to be taught how to notice signs of pain, which is assessed through gentle palpation and manipulation and observation. Demeanor, posture, alertness, eye character, inclination for eating, drinking, elimination, and grooming behaviors, and responses to other ferrets and human family members give clues to the level of discomfort. A ferret in pain has a dull, "haunted" look to their eyes (**Fig. 9**).

The issue becomes one of finding the "right" time for euthanasia. The author considers that when a ferret can no longer maintain itself and/or must be managed on constant, opiate analgesics, that it is time for euthanasia. Owners must be counseled

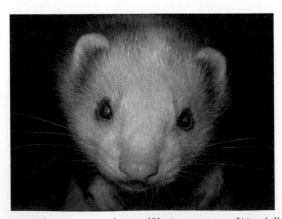

Fig. 8. Bilateral cataracts in a geriatric ferret. (*Photo courtesy of* Vondelle McLaughlin.)

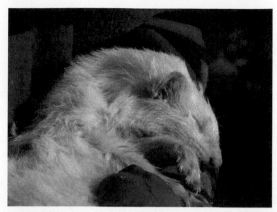

Fig. 9. Dying ferret presented for euthanasia. The ferret was sleeping all the time and refusing food and water.

on how to manage the remaining time, which may give them a chance to say good-bye. The veterinarian can supply the needed medications and nursing care along with a written chart for the owner to follow. This includes instruction on managing pain control and keeping a regular schedule of medications and supportive care. The owners should also be provided a written set of symptoms to look for that indicates a decline in condition. These include: dull eyes, nausea, lack of appetite and/or actively protesting hand feeding, dehydration manifested by skin tenting, sunken eyes, coolness of feet, dry mouth/anus/vulva/prepuce, reluctance to move, vocalizations on handling or moving, black tarry stools, decreased urine or feces, inability to reach the litter tray or move away from eliminations, sleeping 23.5 hours a day and difficulty rousing, consistently lowered body temperature, and cessation of grooming. Gently introducing euthanasia as an alternative to days or weeks of severe pain and complicated medical and supportive therapy when there is no hope of recovery is the veterinarian's compassionate role. Unfortunately, the veterinarian often needs to describe the alternative of "just dying" can include seizures, uncontrolled pain, coldness/fever, bleeding, and loss of control of life and dignity, all of which are traumatic not only to the ferret but to the family members who may observe this. Ferrets are normally joyous animals with a tremendous will to live. It is apparent when this is no longer so: we have to respect their right to maintain happiness and comfort. Although it is extremely difficult to let go, keeping the ferret alive for us rather than for the well-being of the ferret is not the right thing to do. The veterinarian may also provide grief-counselling services.[1]

SUMMARY

The geriatric ferret is likely to present with numerous medical conditions. A program with at least twice-yearly medical evaluations can find problems early and therapy can be initiated. The goal is to allow the ferret maximum longevity with a good quality of life.

DISCLOSURE

The author has nothing to disclose.

REFERENCES

1. Johnson-Delaney CA. Geriatrics. In: Johnson-Delaney CA, editor. Ferret medicine and surgery. Boca Raton (FL): CRC Press; 2017. p. 429–36.
2. Hoppes SM. The senior ferret (*Mustela putorius furo*). Vet Clin Exot Anim 2010;13: 107–22.
3. Malakoff RL, LASTE NJ, Orcutt CJ. Echocardiographic and electrocardiographic findings in client-owned ferrets: 95 cases (1994-2009). J Am Vet Med Assoc 2012;241:1484–9.
4. Morrisey JK, Kraus MS. Cardiovascular and other diseases. In: Quesenberry KE, Carpenter JW, editors. Ferrets, rabbits, and rodents. 3rd edition. St. Louis (MO): W.B. Saunders; 2012. p. 62–77.
5. Morrisey JK, Johnston MS. Ferrets. In: Carpenter JW, Marion CJ, editors. Exotic animal formulary. 5th edition. St. Louis (MO): Elsevier; 2018. p. 532–57.
6. Bakthavatchalu V, Muthupalani S, Marini RP, et al. Endocrinopathy and aging in ferrets. Vet Pathol 2016;53:349–65.
7. Benoit-Blancamano M, Morin M, Langlois I. Histopathologic lesions of diabetes mellitus in a domestic ferret. Can Vet J 2005;46:895–7.
8. Chen A. Pancreatic endocrinopathies in ferrets. Vet Clin Exot Anim Pract 2008;11: 107–23.
9. Hess L. Insulin glargine treatment of a ferret with diabetes mellitus. J Am Vet Med Assoc 2012;241:1490–4.
10. Desmarchelier M, Lair S, Dunn M, et al. Primary hyperaldosteronism in a domestic ferret with an adrenocortical adenoma. J Am Vet Med Assoc 2008;233:1297–301.
11. De Matos RE, Connolly MJ, Starkey SR, et al. Suspected primary hypoparathyroidism in a domestic ferret (*Mustela putorius furo*). J Am Vet Med Assoc 2014; 245:419–24.
12. Chen S, Michels D, Culpepper E. Nonsurgical management of hyperadrenocorticism in ferrets. Vet Clin Exot Anim Pract 2014;17:35–49.
13. Boari A, Papa V, Di Silverio F, et al. Type 1 diabetes mellitus and hyperadrenocorticism in a ferret. Vet Res Commun 2010;34(Suppl 1):108–10.
14. Phair KA, Carpenter JW, Schermerhorn T, et al. Diabetic ketoacidosis with concurrent pancreatitis, pancreatic B islet cell tumor, and adrenal disease in an obese ferret (*Mustela putorius furo*). J Am Assoc Lab Anim Sci 2011;50:531–5.
15. Rosenthal KL, Wyre NR. Endocrine diseases. In: Quesenberry KE, Carpenter JW, editors. Ferrets, rabbits, and rodents. 3rd edition. St. Louis: W.B. Saunders; 2012. p. 86–102.
16. Wagner RA, Piche CA, Jochle W, et al. Clinical and endocrine responses to treatment with deslorelin acetate implants in ferrets with adrenocortical disease. Am J Vet Res 2005;66:910–4.
17. Wagner RA, Finkler MR, Fecteau KA, et al. The treatment of adrenocortical disease in ferrets with 4.7 mg deslorelin acetate implants. J Exot Pet Med 2009; 18:146–52.
18. Petritz OA, Antinoff N, Chen S, et al. Evaluation of portable blood glucose meters for measurement of blood glucose concentration in ferrets (*Mustela putorius furo*). J Am Vet Med Assoc 2013;242:350–4.
19. Watson MK, Cazzini P, Mayer J, et al. Histology and immunohistochemistry of severe inflammatory bowel disease versus lymphoma in the ferret (*Mustela putorius furo*). J Vet Diagn Invest 2016;28:198–206.
20. Long H, di Girolamo N, Selleri P, et al. Polyostotic lymphoma in a ferret (*Mustela putorius furo*). J Comp Path 2016;154:341–4.

21. Papageorgiou S, Gnirs K, Quinton J, et al. Clinical and serologic remission of acquired myasthenia gravis in a domestic ferret (*Mustela putorius furo*). J Am Vet Med Assoc 2019;254:1192–5.
22. Turner PV, Brash ML, Smith DA. Ferrets. In: Pathology of small mammal pets. Hoboken (NJ): John Wiley & Sons, Inc; 2018. p. 89–146.
23. Jones KL, Granger LA, Kearney MT, et al. Evaluation of a ferret-specific formula for determining body surface area to improve chemotherapeutic dosing. Am J Vet Res 2015;76:142–8.
24. van Zealand YRA, Lennoz A, Quinton JR, et al. Prepuce and partial penile amputation for treatment of preputial gland neoplasia in two ferrets. J Small Anim Pract 2015;55:593–6.
25. Vilalta L, Melendez-Lazo A, Canturri A, et al. Anal sac adenocarcinoma with metastases and hypercalcemia in a ferret (*Mustela putorius furo*). J Exot Pet Med 2017;26:143–9.
26. Antinoff N, Williams BH. Neoplasia. In: Quesenberry KE, Carpenter JW, editors. Ferrets, rabbits, and rodents. 3rd edition. St. Louis (MO): W.B. Saunders; 2012. p. 103–21.
27. Schoemaker NJ. Ferret oncology. Diseases, diagnostics, and therapeutics. Vet Clin Exot Anim 2017;20:183–208.
28. Fox-Alvarez WA, Moreno AR, Bush J. Diagnosis and successful surgical removal of an aural ceruminous gland adenocarcinoma in a domestic ferret (*Mustela putorius furo*). J Exot Pet Med 2015;24:350–5.
29. Frohlich JR, Donovan TA. Cervical chordoma in a domestic ferret (*Mustela putorius furo*) with pulmonary metastasis. J Vet Diagn Invest 2015;27:656–9.
30. Fox JG, Muthupalani S, Kupel M, et al. Neoplastic diseases. In: Fox JG, Marini RP, editors. Biology and diseases of the ferret. 3rd edition. Ames: John Wiley & Sons, Inc.; 2014. p. 587–626.
31. Chambers JK, Nakamori T, Kishimoto TE, et al. Lachrymal gland basal cell adenocarcinoma in a ferret (*Mustela putorius furo*). J Comp Path 2016;155:259–62.
32. Eshar D, Wyre NR, Griessmayr P, et al. Diagnosis and treatment of myeloosteolytic plasmablastic lymphoma of the femur in a domestic ferret. J Am Vet Med Assoc 2010;237:407–14.
33. D'Ovidio D, Rossi G, Meomartino L. Oral malignant melanoma in a ferret (*Mustela putorius furo*). J Vet Dent 2016;33:108–11.
34. Kanfer S, Reavill DR. Cutaneous neoplasia in ferrets, rabbits, and guinea pigs. Vet Clin North Am Exot Anim 2013;16:579–98.
35. Miwa Y, Uchida K, Nakayama H, et al. Neuroblastoma of the adrenal gland in a ferret. J Vet Med Sci 2010;72:1229–32.
36. Fisher PG. Exotic mammal renal disease: causes and clinical presentation. Vet Clin North Am Exot Anim Pract 2006;9:33–43.
37. Pollock CG. Disorders of the urinary and reproductive system. In: Quesenberry KE, Carpenter JW, editors. Ferrets, rabbits, and rodents. 3rd edition. St. Louis (MO): W.B. Saunders; 2012. p. 46–61.
38. Vilalta L, Altuzarra R, Molina J, et al. Chylous ascites in 2 ferrets. J Exot Pet Med 2017;26:150–5.
39. Tecilla M, Bielli M, Savarino P, et al. Mesenteric heterotopic ossificans in a ferret (*Mustela putorius furo*): a rare cause of soft tissue ossification. J Exot Pet Med 2018;27:108–12.

Geriatric Care of Rabbits, Guinea Pigs, and Chinchillas

Teresa Bradley Bays, DVM, CVA, DABVP (ECM), CVMMP

KEYWORDS

- Geriatric • Guinea pig • Rabbit • Chinchilla • Pain management • Hospice
- Disease • Alternative therapies

KEY POINTS

- Improved knowledge and resources for care of guinea pigs, rabbits, and chinchillas has led to increased longevity and the need to understand and provide geriatric care in these species.
- Common medical conditions in geriatric small mammal herbivores are described.
- Therapies for pain and medical conditions are described.
- Age is not a disease, and preventative wellness visits and diagnostics are recommended to ensure quality of life for geriatric rabbits, chinchillas, and rabbits.
- Pain management, end of life and hospice care, and euthanasia are discussed.

 Video content accompanies this article at http://www.vetexotic.theclinics.com.

Exotic animal veterinarians should be aware of the unique needs of geriatric patients in those species. Aging is individualized and depends on many variables including diet, environment, genetics, presence of or lack of veterinary care, and exposure to stressful situations. Geriatric animals tend to sleep more, are less active, are more immune suppressed, and are less equipped to handle stressful changes in routine and environment. Age, however, is not a disease, and there are many therapies available to make our patients more comfortable for longer.

Educational resources have improved immensely for exotic companion species, although much of what is available is Internet sourced, including misinformation and information that is not evidence based. However, with pet owners being more educated about diet and husbandry, and more medical resources available to veterinarians, longevity of these species has increased slowly over time (**Table 1**), and longer lifespan makes geriatric diseases more common presentations. With an increasing importance of pets as valued family members, owners of geriatric small mammals are seeking care sooner, as well as more frequently requesting advice

---

Belton Animal Clinic and Exotic Care Center, 1308 North Scott Avenue, Belton, MO 64012, USA
E-mail address: igvet@aol.com

Vet Clin Exot Anim 23 (2020) 567–593
https://doi.org/10.1016/j.cvex.2020.05.006
1094-9194/20/© 2020 Elsevier Inc. All rights reserved.

Table 1
Expected lifespan and approximate age considered to be geriatric for rabbits, guinea pigs, and chinchillas

Species	Expected Life Span	Age Range Commonly Considered Geriatric
Rabbits	7–11 y (up to 12 y*; 18 y is the record[1])	5–6 y
Guinea Pigs	5–8 y (up to 11 y*)	3–6 y
Chinchillas	10–18 y (up to 20 y*)	5–6 y

* In the author's experience.

and guidance for palliative and hospice care in end-of-life stages. This article describes common medical issues seen in and recommendations for caring for geriatric rabbits (*Oryctolagus cuniculus*), guinea pigs (*Cavia porcellus*), and chinchillas (*Chinchilla langeria*).

PHYSICAL EXAMINATIONS

With higher metabolic rates and shorter life spans than most other domestic pets, geriatric small mammal herbivores should have wellness examinations (**Box 1**) more frequently because (1) clients who see their pets daily may not notice subtle, insidious changes until pets are extremely sick; (2) clients may not seek veterinary care during senior years because they associate sleeping more and weight loss as "normal" for geriatric animals; and (3) clients may have the misconception that there is not anything that can be done or that their pet does not have much longer to live.

As guinea pigs, rabbits, and chinchillas age, the incidence of degenerative changes such as arthritis and chronic illnesses such as renal disease and neoplasia become more common (see Common Geriatric Diseases). These medical issues can be detected and treated or managed sooner with examinations done more frequently. Quality of life issues can also be discussed when necessary in order to prepare the owner for eventual scenarios as their pet ages.

Box 1
Wellness examination parameters

Look at the Whole Patient Every Time:
- Check weight at every visit (even for nail trims) and chart to watch for changes
- Watch the patient's affect and demeanor during anamnesis
- While talking to the client observe for posture and mobility issues
- Take a full history including diet and environment and any recent changes
- Do not overlook issues not in presenting complaint
- Perform a full physical examination, every time, looking at the affected part last
- Watch how the patient recovers after the examination

Physical Examination—Additional Areas to Check in Small Mammal Herbivores:
- Auscultation of abdomen for intestinal borborygmus
- Examining mucous membrane color and peripheral circulation by looking at the color of lips, gums, and genitals
- Palpation of the neck and dewlap area
- Oral examination (when possible) using a speculum and light source
- Evaluation of incisors and cheek teeth (sedate or anesthetize if appropriate)
- Palpation of mandible
- Evaluation of the bottoms of feet
- Evaluation of the perianal and perigenital area

Triannual wellness examinations determine current health status, aid in developing a plan to prevent future health problems, and allow follow-up on any preexisting health concerns. Issues are detected earlier, and time is available to reiterate recommendations for husbandry, diet, environment, and enrichment (**Box 2**). The client becomes better educated, and the practitioner can become more familiar with the patient, assess quality of life, diagnose and treat undetected problems, and provide palliative care as necessary.

NUTRITIONAL NEEDS

As small mammal herbivores age, fewer pellets should be fed to limit calorie intake to decrease obesity and promote renal and gastrointestinal health. Increasing grass hay

---

Box 2
Client education handout

Advice for Small Mammal Herbivore Clients with Geriatric Pets
- Weigh pets weekly on a gram scale and keep records
- Learn how to assess body mass and body condition and monitor for changes
- Monitor for behavior changes that could signal health issues such as changes in activity, increased sleeping, lethargy, isolation, not wanting to be handled, or aggression not seen previously
- Monitor stool production and watch for changes in color, consistency, size, and frequency of stools
- Monitor for changes in urine, including amount produced, color, odor, and presence of blood
- Monitor for changes in food or water intake
- Watch for the presence of excess cecotropes (night feces) sticking to the rear end or bottoms of feet
- Watch for changes in posture and mobility
- Watch for increases in drinking and urinating
- Watch for difficulty eating, changes in food preferences (such as not taking normal treats or a decrease in consumption of hay), or dropping food from the mouth
- Watch for changes in hair coat, including dullness, matting, loss of hair
- Monitor for signs of dandruff and severe itchiness
- Monitor for discharge from eyes, nose, or inside ears
- Watch to see if your pet tires easily
- Schedule wellness examinations every 2 to 4 months depending on presence of chronic conditions
- Obtain blood work, urinalysis, and radiographs once or twice per year
- Decrease stress and eliminate changes in environment
- Support nutritionally with syringe feeding formula for herbivores
- Syringe feed warm water twice per day to support kidney function and hydration
- Provide veterinary-prescribed pain medicine as needed and use multimodal therapy when possible
- Provide soft bedding
- Examine feet and perianal/perigenital area daily
- Provide a consistent feeding, exercise, and handling schedule
- Consider alternative modalities when indicated for better quality of life and when other treatments are not helpful (ie, acupuncture, herbs, medical massage, chiropractic)
- Seek veterinary care as soon as problems arise, especially if eating less and less or smaller stools are produced

If any of these changes are noticed or if any changes in behavior from normal are noticed you should seek veterinary care as soon as possible. Not eating/drinking and not defecating or eating/drinking less and defecating less are considered emergencies in rabbits, guinea pigs, and chinchillas—immediately seek the help of a veterinarian with experience in treating exotics. Check the AEMV (Association of Exotic Mammal Veterinarians) Website for veterinary practitioners in your area.

and dark leafy greens while feeding less treats will decrease obesity and aid in maintaining a proper gastrointestinal biome. Geriatric small mammal herbivores may do better if syringe fed herbivore supplement (Critical Care, Oxbow Animal Health, Omaha, NE; Emeraid Herbivore, Lafeber, Cornell, IL) once daily to aid in hydration and ensuring balanced micronutrient content in the diet.

Guinea pigs, rabbits, and chinchillas are grazers, and they eat food with heads in a lowered position. Avoid use of mangers or hay bags that require an arthritic pet to raise its head. Provide food in heavy crocks that cannot be turned over easily. Place food in areas where it cannot be easily contaminated by bedding so it is not inadvertently ingested.

Lacking the hepatic enzyme 1-gulonolactone oxidase needed for the conversion of glucose to ascorbic acid, guinea pigs without supplementation are prone to hypovitaminosis C or scurvy[1] (**Box 3**). Scurvy is painful, affecting joints, exacerbating osteoarthritis, and predisposing those affected to malocclusion, tissue mineralization, pododermatitis, and immune suppression. In patients already chronically deficient in vitamin C, these signs can be seen quickly in sick, stressed, anorexic guinea pigs. Any guinea pig that is hospitalized or boarded should be provided with vitamin C daily to prevent scurvy.

The need for guinea pigs to have 15 mg to 30 mg vitamin C daily[2] becomes more important as they age as absorption and assimilation of nutrients decreases.

Box 3
Signs of scurvy in guinea pigs

- Weakness and lethargy
- Anorexia
- Bruxism
- Weight loss, loss of body condition
- Lameness and mobility issues due to swollen joints
- Unwillingness to move
- Ecchymotic hemorrhages
- Malocclusion
- Petechia on gingiva or bleeding gingiva
- Flaky to ulcerated skin lesions that bleed excessively or do not heal readily
- Pododermatitis
- Tissue mineralization
- Rough hair coat
- Frequent vocalizations due to pain
- Diarrhea
- Recurrent pneumonia or urinary tract infections
- Recurrent dermatophyte or mite infestations due to immune suppression
- Sudden death due to starvation or infection

These signs can be seen in a matter of days in a sick guinea pig that stops eating or eats less that is already suffering a deficiency. Any guinea pig that is hospitalized or boarded should be provided with vitamin C daily to prevent scurvy.

Data from Refs.[8,70,71]

Stabilized vitamin C should be provided in tablet or treat form (Oxbow Natural Science Vitamin C Small Animal Supplement, Oxbow Animal Health, Omaha, NE, USA), or crushed in water and given orally via syringe. Vitamin C in the water bottle or bowl is not recommended, as it may cause the guinea pig to drink less, affecting hydration, renal function, and making urolithiasis more likely. Vegetables high in vitamin C including capsicum, coriander, and tomatoes can be supplemented.

Pellets, fruits, and vegetables, however, do not contain enough vitamin C for daily needs especially if the immune system is challenged. Storage conditions, including exposure to dampness, heat, and light can affect vitamin C potency of pellets within 90 days of milling.[3] Clinical signs are not usually noticed by the client until the guinea pig is really ill (see **Box 3**), so daily supplementation must be stressed as mandatory to the client at every visit.

HYDRATION NEEDS

Rabbits offered diets with hay ad libitum have been found to prefer water bowls over sipper bottles.[4] This preference was not noted in a study involving 10 guinea pigs.[4] The later study inferred that because drinking from sipper bottles in guinea pigs involves jaw movements similar to chewing, guinea pigs may derive a form of behavioral enrichment from sipper bottles to simulate oral processing not being satisfied by the diet.[4]

Both sipper bottles and low-sided, heavy crock water bowls should be provided to geriatric rabbits, guinea pigs, and chinchillas to ensure that they are drinking enough water to maintain hydration. Monitoring water intake is as important in geriatric patients as monitoring food intake. In addition to syringe feeding, warm water could be syringed to older pets on a daily basis to maintain hydration as well as to aid in preventing dehydration of stomach, intestinal, and cecal contents.

A patient with arthritis or neck pain may not be able to reach up to a sipper bottle or may have dental issues that make it difficult to move their tongue to operate a sipper bottle. Placing water bowls and bottles in multiple areas so water is easily reached in shorter trips will also encourage increased drinking. Feeding fresh, dark, leafy greens that are moistened provides additional hydration in a more passive way.

HOUSING NEEDS

Abnormal posturing due to arthritis and obesity may cause senior patients to urinate and defecate in more and different areas making it difficult to establish consistent "potty" areas. Provide litter boxes with lower sides to help them get into and out of the box more easily and use a thinner layer of bedding and straw or hay to help them feel more stable. Providing more boxes that are easier to access will increase success and help to decrease the anxiety. Place litter pans and boxes on the same level of the house or enclosure that the pet spends most of its time.

Tile or wood floors can be very challenging for a pet with mobility issues so provide straw mats, rug runners, bath mats or yoga mats to create better traction. Hay and straw mats are a safe source of fiber and enrichment if they are eaten. Also, provide multiple small, slip resistant steps or a ramp to get up to favored elevated surfaces.

SOCIALIZATION NEEDS

Rabbits and guinea pigs are naturally social creatures and thrive better physically and psychologically in groups of 2 or 3 once bonded. Providing bonded mates for these species is so important psychosocially that Switzerland, a country known for its humane animal legislation, requires by law that guinea pigs be kept at least in pairs in order to decrease stress and anxiety and allow them better quality of life.[5,6]

If one of the bonded mates should pass away it is important to attempt to replace them. The new rabbit or guinea pig should be quarantined and examined by a veterinarian before introduction. Slow, patient, supervised introduction in neutral territory is necessary to minimize fighting. Encourage clients to adopt through the House Rabbit Society or shelter, as they are well versed in introductions and help to find the right mate for the mourning patient.

Chinchillas tend to be more solitary in nature and usually only social during the breeding season. If a bonded mate passes, however, similar attempts to introduce a new mate should be made. Regardless of species, new additions may not get along with already established conspecifics and may eventually have to be housed separately.

GROOMING NEEDS

Many older small mammal herbivores have difficulty grooming themselves due to obesity, arthritis, discospondylosis, undiagnosed musculoskeletal restrictions, and pododermatitis, making it difficult to posture for cleaning and may need to be groomed more frequently. Decreased cognitive function or illness can also contribute to lack of self-grooming.

Care must be taken in handling and positioning arthritic patients for nail trims, perineal cleanings, and grooming. Nails tend to grow more quickly, are thicker, and can curl into foot pads. Guinea pigs, rabbits, and chinchillas that have urine-soaked bottoms should be checked for urinary tract infections, cystic calculi, or calciuria, and they may not be moving as much due to osteoarthritis.

It may become necessary to spot bathe just the perianal area and to monitor for fecal mats, pododermatitis, and urine scalding (see Common Geriatric Issues). Counsel clients to check their pet's bottom and feet daily and clean away any excess urine or fecal matter. House them on substrate that allows urine to wick away from the body to avoid scalding, and perineal areas may need to be clipped periodically to minimize soiling.[7]

Chinchillas need to have access to a dust bath 1 to 2 times per week in order to maintain the integrity or their hair coat. Chinchillas that lack a dust bath or those with musculoskeletal issues that are no longer able to roll in a dust bath, or lack access to a dust bath, develop matted, greasy fur, which may cause them to have decreased ability to thermoregulate.

EXERCISE AND MENTAL STIMULATION

In humans, socialization, exercise, and mental stimulation for geriatric patients help them to live longer with better quality of life and mental acuity. Exercise and mental stimulation in the form of enrichment are important, especially for senior patients. Creating opportunities for moderate exercise, and encouraging play, is essential. Enrichment that provides for making choices in relation to resources, and stimulates exploration and natural behaviors, is important in maintaining physical and mental health. Many resources are available on how to provide enrichment, including Lafebervet.com, Houserabbit.org, and Oxbowanimalhealth.com.

COMMON MEDICAL ISSUES

Senior small mammal herbivores may not recover from illness as readily as their younger conspecifics due to the immune suppression. Weight loss, lethargy, and unthrifty hair coat, however, do not occur because of age but because disease or illness is present. Common medical issues seen in geriatric rabbits, guinea pigs, and chinchillas are described later. Chinchillas, despite having somewhat greater longevity, tend to have fewer medical issues and many are related to deficiencies in husbandry and diet.[1] When treating any of these disease processes it is important to monitor for and treat any secondary gastrointestinal syndrome.

Ocular Disease

Cataracts are common in aging rabbits, guinea pigs, and chinchillas and have multiple causes.[8] *Encephalitozoon cuniculi* is a common cause of cataracts in rabbits with or without phacoclastic uveitis (**Fig. 1**).[7,9] Generally not painful, cataracts may cause patients to be reluctant to move in new surroundings due to decreased visual acuity and changes in depth perception and sensitive to bright light. Cataracts can be treated by phacoemulsification, which may only be necessary if secondary problems such as uveitis and glaucoma occur.

Uveitis and keratitis can be also seen for other reasons in rabbits. Nasolacrimal occlusion is also commonly seen in geriatric rabbits with dental disease, including those with apical overgrowth.[7,8] Resulting dacryocystitis is evidenced by unilateral or bilateral epiphora and can be caused by overgrown roots of cheek teeth and tooth root abscesses.[8] Chronic infections can cause fibrosis of the nasolacrimal duct,[8] and subsequent facial dermatitis occurs from resulting epiphora.

Aged chinchillas are susceptible to posterior cortical cataracts.[10] Asteroid hyalosis, a degenerative condition of the eye involving small white mobile calcium-lipid opacities in the vitreous humor, can also be seen in chinchillas.[10]

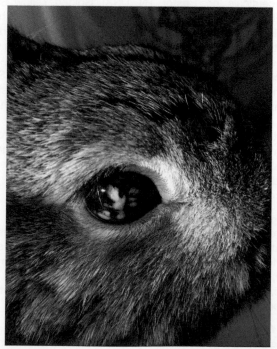

Fig. 1. Phacoclastic uveitis in a geriatric rabbit with *Encephalitozoon cuniculi.*

Chronic Otitis

Chronic otitis can be seen in older lop-eared rabbits and is secondary to stenosis. The severity may necessitate lateral ear canal resection, bulla ostectomy, or total ear canal ablation.[11]

Dermatologic Diseases

Mite infestations

Mite infestations are more commonly noted in geriatric small mammals due to immune suppression, chronic illness, or, in guinea pigs, hypovitaminosis C. Treat ears several times before attempting to clean out the aural debris to decrease pain and stress. Guinea pigs can be so pruritic from mites that they begin to seizure as they scratch and then come up scratching again as the seizure ends (Video 1). Treatment of mites may need to be modified or postponed until an elderly patient is supported and stable.

Pododermatitis

Obesity and decreased mobility, common in geriatric pets, are primary predisposing factors for pododermatitis. Other factors include damp enclosures, lack of exercise, wire or abrasive flooring or substrates, poor nutrition, and urine scalding.[7,8,12] Patients are often reluctant to move, lame, depressed, anorexic, and unable to groom. Resulting abscesses are often attributed to Staphylococcus sp.[1,8] Radiographs are indicated to rule out secondary osteomyelitis.[7,8,12]

Abscesses need to be debrided, flushed, and cultured. Antibiotics and analgesics, along with daily soaking of feet in dilute chlorhexidine solution (Dermachlor Rinse 0.2%, Henry Schein Animal Health, Dublin, OH, USA), is recommended. Azithromycin (Zithromax, Pfizer Inc, NY, USA) at 40 mg/kg q 24 hours PO can be started pending culture and sensitivity results.[1] Silver sulfadiazine cream (SSD, Silvadine Cream 1%, Monarch Pharmaceuticals Inc, Bristol, TN, USA), Golden Yellow Salve (Jing Tang Herbal, Ocala, FL, USA), medical grade honey, or Heal-X Soother Plus Cream (Zoologic Education Network, Lake Worth, FL USA) can be applied topically. Bandages may need to be applied and mole skin can be used to fashion sandals, leaving a center "donut hole" to allow air to get to the debrided lesion. Long-term analgesics including meloxicam (Metacam, Boehringer Ingelheim Vetmedica, St. Joseph, MO, USA) and buprenorphine hydrochloride (Par Pharmaceutical, Chestnut Ridge, NY, USA) are necessary. Other analgesics should be used in patients with renal or hepatic insufficiencies.

Provide softer, thicker bedding; clean and dry enclosure surfaces; restrict calories in overweight patients; and provide vitamin C daily. It takes weeks to months for resolution, and prognosis is poor unless all associated causes are corrected.[7,8,12] Infection extending to tendon, bone, and joints makes the prognosis grave, and amputation may become necessary.[1]

Perianal and perigenital soiling and dermatitis

Geriatric herbivores often present with matted, soiled peri-anal or peri-genital fur with secondary dermatitis. Low-fiber, high carbohydrate diets can lead to soft stools. Urine dribbling from infection, excessive crystalluria, or hypercalciuria may create urine scalding. Obesity, pain, or arthritis may also contribute to decreased ability to groom, to eat cecotropes, and to move away from soiled bedding. Treatment is similar to that listed in the Pododermatitis section.

Impacted scrotal folds and vaginitis

Older, intact, male guinea pigs are prone to impaction of feces, sebum, and bedding in the skin folds associated with the interscrotal septum, which become loose with age

(**Fig. 2**).[1,13] Female guinea pigs can get bedding in the vulva and vaginal vestibule causing irritation and infection.[1] These impactions can become quite large, and gentle cleaning with moistened cotton tipped swabs is needed. Changing bedding to towels or paper towels may be necessary.

Neurologic Disorders

Neurologic diseases in rabbits, guinea pigs, and chinchillas include torticollis, nystagmus, tremors, paresis, paralysis, and seizures.[7] Generally, hyperesthesia can be caused by central or peripheral lesions, whereas seizures and rolling likely indicate central lesions.[14,15] Information on performing a full rabbit neurologic examination and appropriate neurodiagnostics is available for practitioners.[7,16]

Torticollis, most commonly an indication of vestibular dysfunction, can be central, originating from the cerebellum or brain stem, or peripheral, originating from inner ear issues, and was the most common clinical sign noted in a retrospective study of rabbits with neurologic disease.[7,14] Head tilt in rabbits that develops later in life is more likely due to *Encephalitozoon cuniculi*. Hindquarter paresis and/or paralysis and walking instead of hopping with the rear limbs may also be the sequelae to *E cuniculi*. Other vestibular signs include nystagmus and loss of balance and rolling, which can be seen with both otitis interna and infection with *E cuniculi*.

Benzimidazole derivatives have been used to manage and suppress *E.cuniculi* infections in rabbits but have been known to cause a sometimes fatal anemia. This class of drugs has antiinflammatory and in vitro antiprotozoal activity including bioenergetic disruptions of membranes and microtubular inhibition of *E cuniculi*.[7,17,18] *E cuniculi*

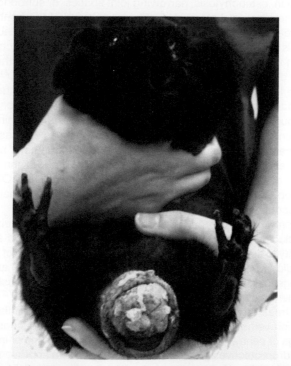

Fig. 2. Older intact male guinea pig with a severe impaction of bedding, sebum, and feces in the perineal/periscrotal skin folds.

has more recently been reclassified from a protozoon to a spore-forming unicellular parasite belonging to the phylum microsporidia so management and treatment is currently being reevaluated.[19]

Management of torticollis includes antibiotic therapy and nutritional supplementation, if appropriate, and environmental support to minimize the rolling and severe ataxia such as providing rolled towels in order to help to keep the patient sternal.[7] Lubricating the eye on the down side of the head tilt is necessary to keep it protected. Treatment with meclizine hydrochloride (Meclizine HCl, Rugby Labs., Duluth GA) can aid in the control of vertigo and rolling. The clinical signs of rolling and nystagmus often resolves but the head tilt may be permanent. Patients with torticollis can live with great quality of life if managed properly (Videos 2 and 3). Management also includes cold laser, medical massage, acupuncture, and veterinary medical manipulation to help with compensatory restrictions.

Musculoskeletal Disease

Osteoarthritis and discospondylosis are commonly encountered in geriatric small mammal herbivores. Inactivity may be inaccurately attributed to advanced age rather than discomfort. Signs of musculoskeletal disease include diminished activity, a hunched posture, varying degrees of paresis, paralysis, stilted gait or lameness, lack of or inability to groom, perineal soiling or dermatitis due to inability to direct the urine stream properly, difficulty getting in and out of the litterbox, no longer using the litterbox, inability to ingest cecotrophs, and altered posturing of limbs when resting or ambulating.

Radiographic evidence of degenerative joint disease and osteoarthritis includes capsular distension, osteophytosis, narrowing joint spaces, or surrounding soft tissue thickening or mineralization. Lateral abduction or splaying of the front limbs may be seen in larger breed senior rabbits due to inactivity and resulting muscle atrophy.[20]

Spondylosis, is an age-related degenerative, noninflammatory condition of the vertebral column with radiographic evidence of osteophytes along the ventral, and/or lateral, and dorsolateral aspects of the vertebral endplates.[21] Found most commonly in the lumbar spine in rabbits, one study indicated that the degenerative change might start as early as 1 year of age during the maturation phase.[21] It is also found, although generally less commonly, in guinea pigs and chinchillas.

Arthritis is a common finding in guinea pigs, can be seen as early as 1 year of age, and is often characterized by superficial fibrillation by 12 months of age and severe cartilage lesions and eburnation as early as 18 months of age.[22] Increasing vitamin C in the diet can assist with inflammation associated with arthritis. Older chinchillas also often develop osteoarthritis and mobility issues along with a change in patterns or routines to accommodate changing locomotor abilities.

An idiopathic progressive osteoarthritis has been documented in guinea pigs[23] with clinical signs including reluctance to move, a hunched position, and a hopping gait. Eventually inability to flex the stifles can occur and bony proliferation of the long bones may be seen radiographically. Histopathology shows a proliferative, ankylosing sclerosis with cartilage loss. Prognosis is poor and the disease is progressive. It has been theorized that there may be an association with hypovitaminosis C.[7,20]

Osteoarthritis treatment is management centered, and pain and inflammation often show marked improvement when treated with analgesics such as nonsteroidal antiinflammatory drugs or centrally acting opiate agonists (**Box 4**) alone or in combination.[7] The use of chondroprotective agents has anecdotally shown improvement in mobility in small mammal herbivores. Pentosan polysulfate sodium, available in Europe and Australasia, has a disease-modifying effect on osteoarthritic joints and is used in

---

Box 4
Analgesics safe for small mammal herbivores

Opiods
- **Buprenorphine** 0.01 to 0.05 mg/kg SC, IM, IV q 6 to 12h; 0.05 mg/kg SC q 8 to 12h
- **Butorphanol** 0.1 to 0.5 mg/kg SC, IM, IV q 2–4h; 1 to 2 mg/kg SC q 4 h (guinea pigs)
- Hydromorphone 0.05 to 0.2 mg/kg SC, IM q 6–8h
- Morphine 2 to 5 mg/kg SC, IM q 4 h
- Oxymorphone 0.1 to 0.5 mg/kg SC, IM q4h
- **Tramadol** 4.4 mg/k IV; 5 to 15 mg/kg PO q8 to 24h
- Meperidine 5-10 mg/kg SC, IM q 2 to 3 h

Nonsteroidal Antiinflammatory Drugs:
- Acetaminophen 200 to 500 mg/kg PO; 1 to 2 mg/mL drinking water
- Acetylsalicylic Acid 100 mg/kg PO q8–24h
- **Carprofen** 2 to 4 mg/kg PO, SC q12 to 24 h
- Ketoprofen 1 to 3 mg/kg SC, IM q12 to 24h
- Piroxicam 0.2 mg/kg PO q8h
- **Meloxicam** 0.1 to 0.3 PO, SC (published doses up to 1 mg/kg PO, SC q24 h)

Neuropathic Analgesia
- **Gabapentin** 3 to 5 mg/kg q 12 to 24h

Visceral and Arthritic pain
- **Maropitant citrate** 2 mg/kg SC q24 h x 3–5d

Drug dosages should be adjusted for the presence of hepatic or renal compromise.

The analgesics that are in bold font are the ones most used by the author.

Data from Refs.[68,72–76]

---

dogs and horses for osteoarthritis and interstitial cystitis.[24] One study indicated that it is also effective as an antiarthritis drug in rabbits.[24] Several joint health products have empirically been found to be safe in small mammal herbivores (**Box 5**).

Other options for osteoarthritis management include cold laser (**Fig. 3**), acupuncture, herbal therapy, veterinary medical manipulation (animal chiropractic), medical massage therapy, and pulsed electromagnetic therapy loops. Weight reduction in obese patients and environmental changes that make food, litterboxes, and water more accessible also helps. Enclosure furniture may need to be lowered, and ramps[12] provided to permit easier accessibility and nonslip, soft bedding should be provided.

Dental Disease

Dental issues in small mammal herbivores are seen at any age and causes include genetics, nutritional secondary hyperparathyroidism associated with a poor diet; trauma; and inadequate calcium, vitamin D, and natural sunlight.[7,20] Molar malocclusions can

---

Box 5
Joint health products that have empirically been found safe for use in small mammal herbivores

Polysulfated glycosaminoglycan (Adequan, American Regent, Inc. Animal Health, Shirley, New York, USA)—2.2 mg/kg SC, IM q3d x 21 to 28 days, then q 14d[77]

Chondroitin sulfate (Cosequin, Nutrimax Laboratories Veterinary Sciences, Lancaster, South Carolina, USA)—use at feline dose[78]

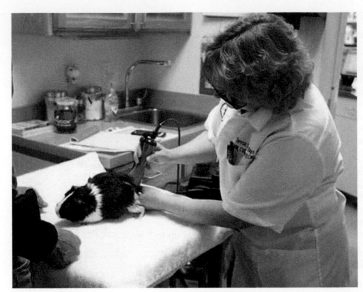

Fig. 3. Cold laser therapy to decrease pain and inflammation and increase blood circulation in a guinea pig with osteoarthritis.

be seen in older rabbits and is most generally caused by tooth root abnormalities such as infection and may also be related to cessation of tooth growth due to attrition of the alveolus.[20]

Malocclusion in guinea pigs causing dental issues is more common in the aged and more prevalent in those with hypovitaminosis C.[1] Temporomandibular joint disorder can occur in senior cavies as the joint becomes weakened allowing the teeth to overgrow. Overstretching during examination and due to elongation of cheek teeth can also stretch the masticatory muscles so that the mouth cannot close properly.

Dental disease is less common in chinchillas but also seen more with age. Subgingival spurs of the upper first, and sometimes second, cheek teeth are commonly missed by practitioners, as a gingivectomy is needed to expose the spurs. Often the only visible sign of this is gingival hyperplasia, sometimes without erythema, at the tooth base with just the occlusal surface of the crown exposed. Both guinea pigs and chinchillas can experience tongue entrapment from overgrown mandibular cheek teeth (**Fig. 4**).

Anesthesia is needed for complete oral examination[7] along with oblique and dorsoventral radiographs of the skull to check crown length, root deformities, and look for periapical abscesses and abnormalities. Patients with dental disease, especially where mandibular abscesses are present, require ongoing dental examination, filing, trimming, and extractions (**Fig. 5**). Antibiotics, if appropriate, and long-term analgesic medication may be needed.[12]

Cardiac Disease

Cardiomyopathy with congestive heart failure, congenital heart defects, myocardial disease, valvular disease, vascular disease, and heart-based neoplasia such as lymphoma and thymoma can occur in rabbits,[25] guinea pigs,[26] and chinchillas.[25] Sustained catecholamine release noted with prolonged stress can induce constriction of coronary vasculature in rabbits resulting in ischemic cardiomyopathy.[27]

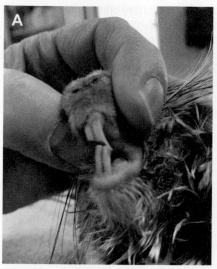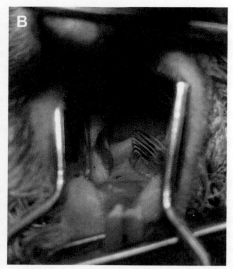

Fig. 4. (*A*) Geriatric chinchilla with malocclusion of incisors. (*B*) Same chinchilla as in Fig. 4a demonstrating lingual points of mandibular cheek teeth overgrowing the tongue causing pain and the inability to eat and drink. Maxillary cheek teeth can be seen with points toward the buccal surfaces.

Diagnosis is made by a combination of clinical signs, radiography, and echocardiography. Signs include exercise intolerance (exhibited by moving less and isolation), coughing, anorexia, depression, increased respiratory rate, dyspnea with exercise, and weight loss.

Despite having smaller than average thoracic space, clinical signs of cardiomegaly, heart disease, and heart-based or mediastinal masses are often not evident until well

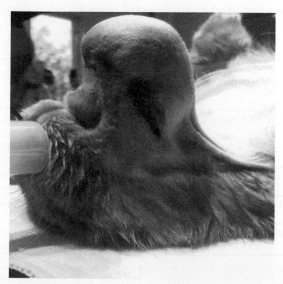

Fig. 5. Mandibular abscess in a geriatric rabbit with periapical infection; note, patient is in dorsal recumbency with its head on the left side of the picture.

into the course of the disease[20] including secondary respiratory compromise in light of pleural effusion, pulmonary infiltration, or cardiomegaly. Symptoms may not be noted until the slowly compromised patient is stressed.[7] Mineralized soft tissue in rabbits and subsequent vascular disease can be secondary to spontaneous arteriosclerosis of the aorta and other major vessels, vitamin D toxicity resulting in calcification of arterial walls and increased afterload, and chronic renal failure.[7,20]

Drugs used to stabilize dogs and cats are used to treat our small mammal herbivores with good result in increasing quality of life and longevity (**Table 2**). Alternative treatments such as acupuncture and herbal therapies also help to keep cardiac patients comfortable for longer.

Respiratory Disease

Chronic respiratory disease is commonly seen in geriatric rabbits and signs include sneezing, nasal discharge, and dacryocystitis secondary to nasolacrimal duct blockage. Underlying stress, poor nutrition, and poor husbandry can predispose elderly patients to bacterial upper respiratory infection or pneumonia often caused by *Pasteurella, Bordetella, Staphylococcus, Streptococcus,* and *Neisseri.*[7,28] It is thought that many rabbits carry *Pasteurella multocida* throughout their lives with no apparent ill effects.[29] Compromise of the immune system can result in latent infection.

Elderly, immune suppressed guinea pigs are susceptible to *Bordetella bronchiseptica* frequently carried by nonsymptomatic rabbits. Other bacteria causing respiratory illness in guinea pigs is cilia-associated respiratory (CAR) *Bacillus* and *Streptococcus pneumonia*, which may also lead to osteoarthritis and cardiac disease.[28] *Streptococcus zooepidemicus* in guinea pigs causes respiratory disease and lymph node abscesses.[1,7]

Immune compromised elderly chinchillas exposed to poor hygiene, poor ventilation, contaminated feed and water, and high humidity may develop respiratory disease. *Pasteurella aeruginosa*, commonly isolated from the gastrointestinal tract of healthy chinchillas, can cause severe respiratory disease in a compromised patient.[10] Cardiac disease should be considered as a differential diagnosis when respiratory signs are present.

Table 2 Drugs used in small mammal herbivores with cardiac disease		
Drug	**Dosage**	**Comments**
Digoxin	0.005–0.01 mg/kg q12–24h	Positive inotropic and antiarrhythmic for CHF, arrhythmias, and DCM
Enalapril	0.5 mg/kg q24–48h PO	ACE inhibitor to dilate vessels for CHF, hypertension, and decrease urine protein loss
Furosemide	1–4 mg/kg q4–6h PO	Loop diuretic to decrease edema in CHF, liver and kidney disease, and treat hypertension
Pimobendan	0.1–0.3 mg/kg q12–24h PO	Positive inotropic and vasodilator for CHF due to DCM or mitral valve disease
Taurine	100 mg/kg q24 h PO	Improves cardiac function in rabbits with artificially induced heart failure

Drug dosages should be adjusted for the presence of hepatic or renal compromise.
Abbreviations: ACE, angiotension-converting enzymes; CHF, congestive heart failure; DCM, dilated cardiomyopathy.
Data from Refs.[27,79,80]

Renal Disease

Chronic renal disease is commonly seen in small mammal herbivores with clinical signs, including dehydration, anorexia, weight loss, polyuria, polydipsia, dull hair coat, failure to groom, diarrhea, and lethargy.[20,30] One postmortem study found histologic lesions of renal disease in 32.5% of 237 rabbits found dead or euthanized because of illness and in 25% of 77 apparently healthy adult rabbits.[31]

Causes include hypervitaminosis D, hydronephrosis, renal agenesis, renal cysts, bacterial infection, neoplasia, nephrocalcinosis, and nephroliths.[7,30,31] E cuniculi in rabbits can cause chronic interstitial nephritis[7,32,33] due to damage caused by the organism. Undetected, chronic, low-grade dehydration should also be considered in patients fed mostly pellets. Diagnosis is based on presence of azotemia, often with hyperphosphatemia and nonregenerative anemia.[33]

Progression is measured by changes in urinalysis parameters (proteinuria, hematuria, and glucosuria) and azotemia, which is detected later in the disease.[8,12] Supportive care includes fluid administration, antibiotics, and erythropoietin injections[30] (Epogen, Amgen, Thousand Oaks, CA, USA), if indicated.

SEGMENTAL NEPHROSCLEROSIS IN GUINEA PIGS

An incidental finding, this segmental interstitial renal scarring is found at necropsy in guinea pigs older than 1 year. Cause is unknown but consideration has been made for an association with high protein diets, autoimmune diseases, infectious diseases, and focal ischemia and fibrosis resulting from vascular disease.[34] Advanced cases may cause azotemia, isosthenuria, and nonregenerative anemia. Metastatic mineralization may be seen in muscle, heart, lungs, foot pads, gastrointestinal system, and corneas.[7,35]

Hyperthyroidism in Guinea Pigs

Hyperthyroidism is underdiagnosed in geriatric guinea pigs and was an incidental necropsy finding in a study of 19 that died from other reasons.[36] Eight of them were benign thyroid hyperplasia and 11 had malignant thyroid adenocarcinoma.[36] Signs are associated with increased metabolic rate and include hyperactivity, weight loss despite voracious appetite, hyperactivity, tachycardia, soft stools, polyuria, and polydipsia.[37] Diagnosis is based on blood work or postmortem findings. Nuclear scintigraphy can help to obtain a more definitive diagnosis but is an expensive diagnostic choice.[36] Treatment consists of oral antithyroid medication or radioactive treatment with I-131.[37]

Metastatic Calcification in Guinea Pigs

Metastatic calcification, or organ mineralization, has been seen primarily in older male guinea pigs with calcium deposits occurring in the gastrointestinal tract, skeletal muscles, joints, lungs, and visceral organs.[38] Often asymptomatic, clinical signs include joint stiffness, weight loss, renal failure, and sudden death.[1,39] Diets high in calcium and phosphorus and low in magnesium and potassium are implicated in the cause, and it is therefore not commonly seen in guinea pigs on diets that mainly include grass hays and green leafy vegetables.[1]

Reproductive Diseases

Reproductive conditions are common in intact geriatric small mammal herbivores. A serosanguinous vaginal discharge is often the first clinical sign observed and patients present due to "bloody urine." Differential diagnoses include porphyria, urolithiasis, and cystitis. Frank blood in the urine due to reproductive disorders is most obvious as blood clots at the end of micturition, whereas, hematuria due to cystitis, renal, or ureteral issues is evidenced by blood in and throughout micturition. Cystic mammary glands and cystic ovaries may develop concurrently with uterine disease. In advanced stages, depression, anorexia, ascites, dyspnea, and severe anemia can be seen.[40]

Rabbits

The most common age-related reproductive issues in rabbits are uterine adenocarcinoma and endometrial hyperplasia, or uterine polyps, resulting in cystic and hyperplastic changes in the endometrial glands.[41] Diagnosis is made by clinical signs of lethargy, anemia, and intermittent hematuria; palpation of firm irregular uterus; and imaging such as radiographs, ultrasound, and computed tomography. Differential diagnoses for uterine enlargement include pregnancy, pyometra, metritis, hydrometra, mucometra, endometrial venous aneurysms, endometrial hyperplasia, leiomyosarcoma, or other neoplasia.[40,41]

Incidence of uterine adenocarcinoma is reported as high as 60% to 80% in does older than 3 years with Tan, French Silver, Havana, and Dutch breeds having a higher incidence[42,43] and can occur despite breeding history.[43] With age the endometrium undergoes a progressive decrease in cellularity and an increase in collagen content leading to a continuum of change from uterine polyp formation to cystic endometrial hyperplasia, adenomatous hyperplasia, and adenocarcinoma and is caused by senile atrophy of the endometrium.[41]

Metastasis to the lungs, liver, brain, and bones occurs via hematogenous spread within 1 to 2 years.[41,44] In breeding does, clinical signs include decreased fertility, fetal resorption, and stillbirths.[40] Other associated conditions, more common in older rabbits, include mammary adenocarcinoma, uterine leiomyoma and leiomyosarcomas, squamous cell carcinoma of the vaginal wall, cystic mastitis, and pyometra.[43]

Ovariohysterectomy (OVH) is the treatment of choice and curative early in the disease. Radiographs to screen for pulmonary metastasis can serve as a prognostic indicator. Affected rabbits should be evaluated and radiographed every 3 to 4 months for 2 years postsurgery for evidence of abdominal or pulmonary metastasis. Encourage clients to spay does before 9 months of age.[40,41]

Guinea pigs

Neoplasia, cystic ovaries, pyometra, and hydrometra are common in intact female guinea pigs older than three years, with an incidence as high as 77% in sows older than 6 years.[45,46] Disorders of the vagina of guinea pigs were found to be rare and included leiomyoma, polyps, and vaginitis.[46] Uterine disorders, however, were diagnosed in 17.4% of full postmortem examinations and 98.1% of the uterine biopsy samples.[45]

Ovarian cysts are spontaneously formed, nonfunctional, fluid-filled cysts near the ovaries[46] (Fig. 6). Cause is unknown, but exposure to estrogenic substances, obesity, and hormonal imbalances are implicated. Many are derived from the rete ovarii but may also occur due to periovarian structures, overgrown Graafian follicles, neoplasia, and infection.[47] Reproductive history has not been found to alter the prevalence of cyst formation.[48] Advancing age does correlate however with increase in size and prevalence of the cysts.[48]

A study in 2003, at a large guinea pig breeding facility, indicated that 58% of sows had ovarian cysts, 38% with bilateral involvement.[48] Unilateral cysts are more commonly seen in the right ovary.[48] Sows older than 18 months had an 88% incidence of cysts with 4.7% showing signs of symmetric dorsal and flank, nonpruritic

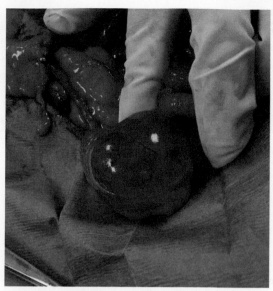

Fig. 6. Ovarian cyst in a geriatric guinea pig. The cysts can be of various sizes.

alopecia.[48] Another study from 2002 observed a 22.4% prevalence of follicular cysts in normal cycling sows.[49] In a study of 655 postmortem guinea pig cases, 245 were found to have ovarian cysts (37.4%) and 38 of 43 ovarian biopsy samples (88.4%).[45]

Caudal abdominal distention and discomfort may be noted along with anorexia, lethargy, and pancytopenia.[38] Acute presentations may occur if ovarian cyst become extremely large,[40] often with secondary gastrointestinal syndrome, and ovarian cysts can become abscessed (**Fig. 7**). Radiographs are not always diagnostic, due to the superimposition of the gastrointestinal tract, and abdominal ultrasonography or exploratory may be required for definitive diagnosis.

Medical therapy has been attempted using short-acting GnRH agonists (Cystorelin Merial, Duluth GA, USA),[50,51] hCG, leuprolide,[40] with limited success.[51] Also, the deslorelin-containing implant Suprelorin (Virbac Veterinary Medicine GmbH, Germany) was studied in a group of 11 nulliparous sows with ovarian cysts and no significant size change of the cyst was noted up to 16 weeks postimplantation.[51]

Ultrasound-guided percutaneous drainage can provide rapid improvement, but recurrence is likely without surgery.[13,38] OVH is the treatment of choice for ovarian cysts. More recently flank ovariectomy with or without complete hysterectomy has been advocated, but consideration for complete OVH should be given to the fact that ovarian cysts have been associated with several uterine diseases including leiomyoma, granulosa cell tumors, endometritis, and cystic endometrial hyperplasia.[7,13,47]

Chinchillas
Most reproductive system disorders found in chinchillas are not age dependent with the exception of endometritis, which, as in rabbits, is likely associated with senile atrophy of the endometrium.

Neoplasia

Occurrence of neoplasia and types of neoplasia represented vary significantly between species and incidence is likely to increase with age. Those more commonly seen in geriatric rabbits, guinea pigs, and chinchillas are listed in the following section.

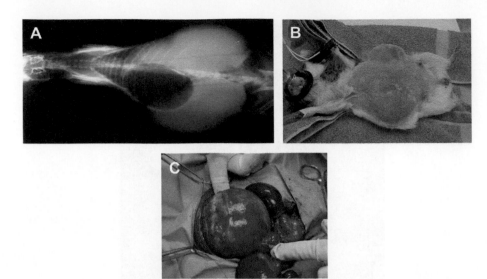

Fig. 7. (A) Ventrodorsal radiograph of an elderly guinea pig with severely enlarged ovarian masses; note, cranial is to the left in the radiograph. (B) Same guinea pig as Fig. 7A during prep for surgery. (C) Intraoperative photo of abscessed cystic ovaries found during exploratory of the guinea pig in Fig. 7A.

Rabbits

Uterine adenocarcinoma is the most commonly seen neoplasm in rabbits. The author recommends that all female rabbits have an OVH performed, preferably before 6 months of age, to prevent occurrence. Older intact female rabbits, after imaging to rule out metastasis, should also be considered candidates for OVH, in order to extend longevity and quality of life.

Thymic neoplasia can also affect older rabbits. The thymus of rabbits is large and persists into adulthood in rabbits. Thymoma is a slow growing, locally invasive benign neoplasm of thymic epithelial cells and is usually composed of lymphoid and reticular epithelial cells.[52,53] No apparent sex predilection exists and mean age is 6 to 7 years.[52–54] Thymic lymphoma, a less commonly occurring malignant neoplasia, involves the lymphoid component of the thymus and is T-lymphocytic origin (**Fig. 8**).[53]

Clinical signs of mediastinal masses, often not detected early in the disease, include nostril flaring, tachypnea, dyspnea, open mouth breathing,[20,52] exercise intolerance, anorexia, and lethargy. Bilateral exophthalmos and prolapse of the third eyelid can occur due to pooling of blood in the retrobulbar venous plexus secondary to cranial vena caval compression (**Fig. 9**). Impaired venous return to the heart may cause edema of the head, neck, and forelimbs.[52] Compression of the heart may result in a heart murmur.[52]

Diagnosis is made by ultrasonic-guided aspiration cytology or biopsy, computed tomography with contrast, or MRI. Thoracotomy to dissect out the tumor may offer the best chance for a cure but is accompanied by surgical risks and postoperative complications. In general, radiation therapy has shown greater long-term success with fewer side effects than chemotherapy.[53–57] Aspiration of cystic fluid may increase quality of life by reducing dyspnea.[55]

Paraneoplastic syndromes in rabbits include hemolytic anemia and exfoliative dermatitis with sebaceous adenitis.[58] Paraneoplastic hyercalcemia[59] was described in 5 of 19 thymoma cases in a retrospective study.[54] The author has had great success

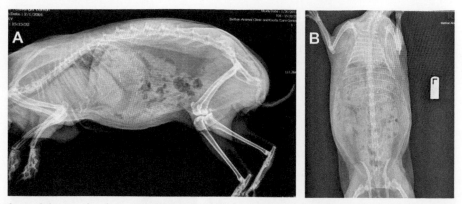

Fig. 8. (*A*) Lateral radiograph of geriatric rabbit with thymic lymphoma presented for severe dyspnea. (*B*) Ventrodorsal radiograph of the same rabbit with thymic lymphoma.

increasing quality of life and longevity in 2 thymic lymphoma rabbits using conventional treatment along with acupuncture and a Chinese herb (Stasis Breaker, Jing Tang Herbal, Reddick, FL, USA) (**Fig. 10**).

Guinea pigs
Guinea pigs tend to have a lower incidence of neoplasia than many small mammals but risk increases when older than 3 years.[60] Reproductive tumors occur most

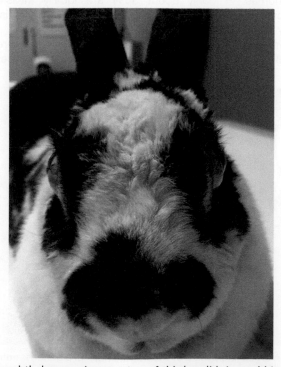

Fig. 9. Bilateral exophthalmos and protrusion of third eyelids in a rabbit due to thymoma. (*Photo courtesy of* Vicki Johnson, DVM.)

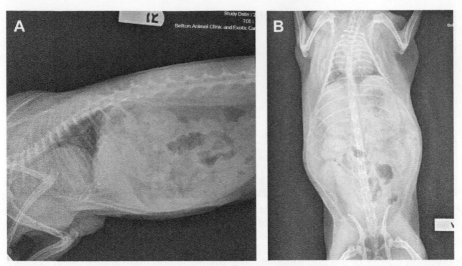

Fig. 10. (*A, B*) Lateral and ventrodorsal radiographs of the same rabbit in **Fig. 8** after 2 months of treatment with prednisone, famotidine, aqua acupuncture, and the Chinese herb combination Stasis Breaker. The dyspnea had resolved, and the rabbit lived comfortably for a year after the diagnosis was made.

commonly in the uterus, and the uterine leiomyoma (**Fig. 11**) is the most common.[61] Mammary tumors can be seen in both male and female guinea pigs, and most are benign fibroadenomas.[62,63] Only about 30% are locally invasive adenocarcinomas.[62,63] The ovarian teratoma occurs in sows older than 3 years, is commonly unilateral, and rarely metastasizes.[60]

The most common skin tumor found in 2 studies in guinea pigs were trichofolliculomas (45% and 38%, respectively[64]), benign tumors of the hair follicles often found in

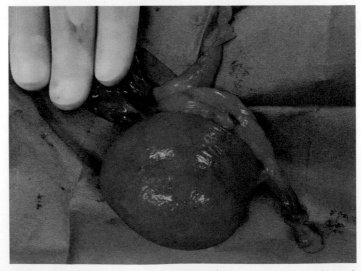

Fig. 11. Severely enlarged leiomyoma of the uterine horn in a geriatric guinea pig that lived for 2 years postsurgery.

cavies older than 3 years. They occur mostly in males and usually on the dorsum, lateral trunk, and lateral thighs.[1] These tumors frequently ulcerate, rupture, and contain caseous debris. Surgical excision is the treatment of choice.

Chinchillas

Although chinchillas live relatively longer than most small mammals, neoplasia is not a common finding,[60] and a retrospective study of 325 chinchillas presented at a university veterinary hospital from 1994 to 2003 indicated that only 1% had evidence of neoplasia.[10] Tumors reported include malignant lymphoma, neuroblastoma, uterine leiomyosarcoma carcinoma, lipoma, hepatic carcinoma, lumbar osteosarcoma, and adenocarcinoma of the lung.[1,10]

COGNITIVE DYSFUNCTION

Signs of senility include isolation, vocalizing at inappropriate times, staring into space, and difficulty remembering routines. Sight and hearing may also be impaired but with senility the ability to navigate well may be more affected by memory and cognitive changes. Eye-blink classical conditioning, used in the study of memory, learning, and brain aging, is impaired in aging rabbits and humans.[65] Rabbits are used for testing cognition-enhancing drugs and in preclinical trials for testing drugs for human patients with Alzheimer disease.[65,66]

Exercise, mental stimulation, consistent routine, social interaction, and good nutritional plane can help to limit signs of senility. Maintaining consistency in the location of enclosure furniture, food, and toys may be helpful for those whose cognitive abilities and sight are impaired. Exercise and enrichment provided throughout life, and continued through geriatric years, can help to stem signs of cognitive dysfunction.

MANAGEMENT OF PAIN, MOBILITY ISSUES, AND CHRONIC DISEASES

Assessing pain in small mammal herbivores and other prey species can be difficult, as natural behavior is to hide signs until too sick to pretend anymore. Signs of pain are also often very subtle and insidious making them more difficult to recognize.

Clinical signs include reluctance to move, vocalizations, bruxism, abdominal pressing, inability to ambulate correctly, fecal and urine matting, unkempt coat, lameness and stiffness, lethargy, vocalizations, strained facial expression with bulging eyes, over grooming or chewing at the affected area, stinting on palpation, arched back, elevated respiratory rate, piloerection, and head held up and extended outward.[67,68] Patients that become aggressive, isolate themselves, or that no longer want to be handled may do so because of undiagnosed pain and restriction.

There are many safe medications and many alternative modalities that allow pets to live more comfortably for longer (see **Box 5**). Incorporating an integrative approach of eastern modalities along with western medications can allow for second chances to many geriatric patients. Holistic and alternative therapies include cold laser therapy, acupuncture, herbal therapy, pulsed electromagnetic therapy loops, medical massage, veterinary medical manipulation, and various forms of electrical stimulation and microcurrent electrical therapy. It is important to discuss expectations for therapies used with goals to make patients more comfortable, less anxious, and to improve quality of life.

GRIEVING THE LOSS OF A BONDED COMPANION

For rabbits and guinea pigs the death of a bonded mate can cause a significant grief response that may be evidenced by isolation, lethargy, eating less, and aggression and biting that had not been previously noted. Also, singly kept pets are especially prone to anxiety and stress created by loss of a bonded caregiver[68] so it is important to make sure that an alternate caregiver be one the pet has been exposed to previously. Spending more time with the pet that is mourning, and providing interaction and enrichment, can help.

Clients should check local rescue groups to find new companions. Proper quarantine, veterinary examinations, and intestinal parasite examinations for the new pet should be done before introduction. Adult-supervised, gradual introductions in neutral territory are necessary to minimize fighting, and consideration should be made that the new pair or trio will not bond and may require separate spaces or enclosures.

HOSPICE CARE

The need to guide clients to provide hospice care for their pets is becoming more common. Providing comfort and controlling pain and anxiety are hospice goals. An individual plan of medical and alternative therapies should be developed for the unique circumstances of each pet. Making clear recommendations and providing clear expectations is important in communicating well with clients who wish to care for their dying pets at home.

Syringing food and water may become necessary, but encourage clients to never force a pet to eat, which may cause anxiety or potential aspiration. Counsel clients that at some point their pet will stop eating, near end of life, and organs will not function well. Choose bedding that is easily cleaned and changed. Maintaining hygiene is important to prevent decubital ulcers, urine scalding, and infections. Shaving the hair from these areas will keep the skin dry and aid in cleaning, although rabbits should not have the bottoms of their feet shaved. Ophthalmic lubricants may become necessary to keep patients comfortable.

QUALITY-OF-LIFE CONSIDERATIONS

There have not been any resources developed for small mammal herbivores to help to make quality-of-life decisions, but in general lack of appetite, severe mobility restrictions, pain that cannot be controlled, and a lack of response to owner interaction may be used.[7] **Box 6** provides resources that have been developed for dogs and cats in order to help caregivers to determine quality of life and aid in making end-of-life decisions.

EUTHANASIA

Minimize stress, fear, and anxiety before and during euthanasia. The author prefers to anesthetize small mammal patients after sedation.[12,69] An injection of euthanasia solution is then given intravenously using a small gauge butterfly catheter or via intracardiac administration. The clients are then allowed to be with the deceased pet if they wish.

Have the client sign for, decide on after care, and pay for the euthanasia before the procedure. Ask if they would like a swatch of fur or paw print before the procedure. Information on grief counseling and local counselors can be passively provided along with the paid invoice so that grieving clients can reach out for help if needed. Allow them to spend as much time with their pet before and after death as they need.

Afterward escort them through a private way out of the building so that they do not have to go through the lobby while grieving. Send a sympathy card signed by staff and an ink or clay paw print soon after the appointment. Consider making a donation to the

---

Box 6
Resources for owners to make quality-of-life and end-of-life decisions

- *Pet Quality of Life Scale*: Pet Quality of Life Scale and Daily Diary by Dr Gardner[81]

- *Good Days versus Bad:* track the days when your pet is feeling good as well as the days when he or she is not feeling well, and using a check mark for good days and an X for bad days on your calendar can help you determine when a loved one is having more bad days than good.[82] The Gray Muzzle application developed by 2 veterinarians, Drs Gardner and McVety,[81] and produced by their Lap of Love Veterinary Hospice has a calendar so clients can visualize the month at a glance as well as a summary page to see a pie chart of their pet's progress or decline.

- *The Rule of "Five Good Things":* pick the top 5 things that the pet loves to do. When he or she can no longer do 3 or more of them, quality of life has been affected to a level where many veterinarians might recommend euthanasia.[82]

- *HHHHHMM:* Dr Alice Villalobos is a well-known veterinary oncologist who created the "HHHHHMM" Quality of Life Scale. The anacronym stands for Hurt, Hunger, Hydration, Happiness, Hygiene (the ability to keep the pet clean from bodily waste), Mobility, and More (more good days than bad). Grade each category on a scale of 1 to 10, with 1 being poorest quality of life and 10 being best. If most of the categories are ranked as 5 or higher, continuing with supportive care is considered acceptable.[82]

- *Pet Hospice Journal:* keeping a journal of your pet's condition, behavior, appetite, etc., can be extremely valuable in evaluating quality of life over time.[82]

---

local House Rabbit Society or rescue group for that species in the name of that pet and reference it in the sympathy card.

SUPPLEMENTARY DATA

Supplementary data related to this article can be found online at https://doi.org/10.1016/j.cvex.2020.05.006.

REFERENCES

1. Jenkins J. Diseases of geriatric guinea pigs and chinchillas. Vet Clin North Am Exot Anim Pract 2010;13(1):85–93.

2. Harkness JE, Turner PV, VandeWoude S, et al. Harkness and Wagner's biology and medicine of rabbits and rodents. 5th ediiton. Hoboken (NJ): Wiley-Blackwell; 2010.

3. Cheeke PR. Rabbit feeding and nutrition; Chapter 19 – nutrition of Guinea pigs. Orlando (FL): Academic Press, Inc; 1987. p. 349.

4. Balsiger A, Clauss M, Liesegang A, et al. Guinea pig (Cavia porcellus) drinking preferences: do nipple drinkers compensate for behaviourally deficient diets? J Anim Physiol Anim Nutr (Berl) 2017;101(5):1046–56.

5. Andrei M. "Why it's illegal to own one guinea pig in Switzerland" 4-10-16 with update 5-30-18. Available at: www.zmescience.com. Accessed September 21, 2019.

6. Available at: https://www.techly.com.au/2016/03/14/in-switzerland-its-illegal-to-own-just-one-guinea-pig-due-to-loneliness/. Accessed October 12, 2019.

7. Fisher PG. Exotic Mammal Geriatrics. Western Veterinary Conference. Las Vegas (NV), February 20–24, 2011.

8. Rosenthal KL. How to Manage the Geriatric Rabbit. Atlantic Coast Veterinary Conference;. Atlantic City (NJ): October 9-11, 2001.

9. Csokai J, Joachim A, Gruber A, et al. Diagnostic markers for encephalitozoonosis in pet rabbits. Vet Parasitol 2009;163(1–2):18–26.

10. Available at: www.merckveterinarymanual.com, veterinary/exotic and laboratory animals/rodents/chinchillas Donnelly TM. Accessed September 21, 2019.

11. Capello V. Surgical treatment of otitis externa and media in pet rabbits. Exotic DVM 2004;6(3):15.

12. Carmel B. The Elder Rabbit: Care and Welfare of the Geriatric Pet Rabbit. Proceedings Australian Veterinary Association. Sunny Hills (N.S.W), June, 2010.

13. Harcourt-Brown F. Urogenital diseases. In: Harcourt-Brown F, editor. Textbook of rabbit medicine. London: Elsevier Science Limited; 2002. p. 335–51.

14. Gruber A, Pakozdy A, Weissenböck H, et al. A retrospective study of neurological disease in 118 rabbits. J Comp Pathol 2009;140:31–7.

15. Harcourt-Brown F. Neurological and locomotor disorders. In: Harcourt-Brown F, editor. Textbook of rabbit medicine. Oxford (United Kingdom): Butterworth-Heinemann; 2002. p. 307–23.

16. Vernau KM, Osofsky A, LeCouteur RA. The neurological examination and lesion localization in the companion rabbit (Oryctolagus cuniculus). Vet Clin North Am Exot Anim Pract 2007;10:731–58.

17. Suter C, Muller-Doblies UU, Hatt JM, et al. Prevention and treatment of Encephalitozoon cuniculi infection in rabbits with fenbendazole. Vet Rec 2001;148:478–80.

18. Franssen FF, Lumeij JT, van Knappen F. Susceptibility of Encephalitozoon cuniculi to several drugs in vitro. Antimicrob Agents Chemother 1995;39:1265–8.

19. Bohne W, Bottcher K, Gross U. The parasitophorous vacuole of *Encephalitozoon cuniculi*: biogenesis and characteristics of the host cell-pathogen interface. Int J Med Microbiol 2011;301(5):395–9.

20. Lennox AM. Care of the geriatric rabbit. Vet Clin North Am Exot Anim Pract 2010; 13(1):123–33.

21. Leung VYL, Hung SC, Wu EX, et al. Age-related degeneration of lumbar intervertebral discs in rabbits revealed by deuterium oxide-assisted MRI. Osteoarthritis Cartilage 2008;16:1312–8.

22. McKCiombor D, Aaron RK, Wang S, et al. Modification of osteoarthritis by pulsed electromagnetic field—a morphological study. Osteoarthritis Cartilage 2003;11: 455–62.

23. Gurkan I, Ranganathan A, Yang X, et al. Modification of osteoarthritis in the guinea pig with pulsed low-intensity ultrasound treatment. Osteoarthritis Cartilage 2010;18(5):724–33.

24. Smith MM, Ghosh P, Numata Y, et al. The effects of orally- administered calcium pentosan polysulphate on inflammation and cartilage degradation produced in rabbit joints by intraarticular injection of a hyaluronate polylysine complex. Arthritis Rheum 1994;37(1):125–36.

25. Heatley JJ. Small exotic mammal cardiovascular disease. Proceedings Association of Exotic Mammal Veterinarians Scientific Program. Providence (RI), August 5, 2007.

26. Cox I, Haworth P. Cardiac disease in guinea pigs. Vet Rec 2000;146(21):620.

27. Pariaut R. Cardiovascular physiology and diseases of the rabbit. Vet Clin North Am Exot Anim Pract 2009;12:135–44.

28. Schoeb TR. Respiratory diseases of rodents. Vet Clin North Am Exot Anim Pract 2000;3(2):481–96.

29. Harcourt-Brown F. Cardiorespiratory disease. In: Harcourt-Brown F, editor. Textbook of rabbit medicine. Melbourne (Australia): Butterworth-Heinemann; 2002. p. 324–34.

30. Pare JA, Paul Murphy J. Disorders of the reproductive tract and urinary systems. In: Quseberry KE, Carpenter JW, editors. Ferrets, rabbits and rodents, clinical medicine and surgery. St Louis (MO): Saunders; 2004. p. 183–93.

31. Hinton M. Kidney disease in the rabbit: a histological survey. Lab Anim 1981;15: 263–5.

32. Csokai J, Grube A, Kunzel F, et al. Encephalitozoonosis in pet rabbits (Oryctolagus cuniculus): pathological findings in animals with latent infection versus clinical manifestation. Parasitol Res 2009;104(3):629–35.

33. Wong C. Diet and acute renal failure in rabbits. Clinician's Brief, Urology and Nephrology. Tulsa (OK): Brief Media; 2007.

34. Percy DN, Barthold SW. Guinea pig. In: Pathology of laboratory rabbits and rodents. 3rd edition. Ames (IA): Blackwell Publishing; 2007. p. 217–52.

35. Garner M, Johnson-Delaney C. Diseases of cavies. Proceedings of the Association of Avian Veterinarians. Savannah (GA), August 10, 2008.

36. Gibbons P, Garner M. Pathological aspects of thyroid tumors in guinea pigs (Cavia porcellus). Proceedings of the Association of Exotic Mammal Veterinarians. Milwaukee (WI). 2009: p. 81.

37. Mayer J, Wagner R. Clinical aspects of hyperthyroidism in the guinea pig. Proceedings of the Association of Exotic Mammal Veterinarians, Milwaukee (WI), August 12–15, 2009.

38. O'Rourke DP. Disease problems of guinea pigs. In: Quesenberry KE, Carpenter JW, editors. Ferrets, rabbits and rodents clinical medicine and surgery. Philadelphia: Saunders; 2004. p. 245–54.

39. Holcombe H, Parry NM, Rick M, et al. Hypervitaminosis D and metastatic calcification in a colony of inbred strain 13 guinea pigs, cavia porcellus. Vet Pathol 2015;52(4):741–51.

40. Johnson DJ. Reproductive Tract Tumors and Diseases in Exotic Companion Mammals. American Board of Veterinary Practitioners. Glendale (AZ), October 31–November 3, 2013.

41. Klaphake E, Paul-Murphy J. Disorders of the reproductive and urinary systems. In: Queseberry K, Carpenter J, editors. Ferrets, rabbits and rodents: clinical medicine and surgery. 3rd ediiton. St Louis (MO): Elsevier; 2012. p. 217–31.

42. Ritzman T. Small mammal neoplasia. Proceedings CVC, San Diego (CA). October 1, 2008.

43. Heatley J, Smith A. Spontaneous neoplasms of lagomorphs. Vet Clin North Am Exot Anim Pract 2004;7(3):561–77.

44. Grant A. Exotic animal geriatrics. In: Gardner M, McVety D, editors. Treatment and care of the geriatric veterinary patient. Hoboken (NJ): Wiley Blackwell; 2017. p. 245–55.

45. Bertram CA, Müller K, Klopfleisch R. Genital tract pathology in female pet guinea pigs (Cavia porcellus): a retrospective study of 655 post-mortem and 64 biopsy cases. J Comp Pathol 2018;165:13–22.

46. Pilny A. Ovarian cystic disease in guinea pigs. Vet Clin North Am Exot Anim Pract 2014;17(1):69–75.

47. Bean A. Ovarian cysts in the guinea pig. Vet Clin North Am Exot Anim Pract 2013; 16(3):757–76.

48. Nielson TD, Holt S, Ruelokke ML, et al. Ovarian cyst in guinea pigs: influence of age and reproductive status on prevalence and size. J Small Anim Pract 2003;44: 257–60.

49. Shi F, Petroff BK, Herath CB, et al. Serous cysts are a benign component of the cyclic ovary in the guinea pig with an incidence dependent upon inhibin bioactivity. J Vet Med Sci 2002;64(2):129–35.

50. Mayer J. The use of GnRH to treat cystic ovaries in a Guinea pig. Exotic DVM 2003;5(5):36.

51. Schuetzenhofer G, Goericke-Pesch S, Wehrend A. Effects of deslorelin implants on ovarian cysts in guinea pigs. Schweiz Arch Tierheilkd 2011;153(9):416–7.

52. Künzel F, Hittmair K, Hassan J, et al. Thymomas in rabbits: clinical evaluation, diagnosis, and treatment. J Am Anim Hosp Assoc 2012;48(2):97–104.

53. Graham J. Rabbit thymoma vs lymphoma: diagnostic and therapeutic options. Michigan Veterinary Medical Association. Lansing (MI), January 26–28, 2018.

54. Andres K, Kent M, Siedlecki C, et al. The use of megavoltage radiation therapy in the treatment of thymomas in rabbits: 19 cases. Vet Comp Oncol 2012;10(2): 82–94.

55. Huston S, Lee P, Quesenberry K, et al. Cardiovascular disease, lymphoproliferative disorders, and thymomas. In: Quesenberry KE, Carpenter JW, editors. Ferrets, rabbits, and rodents: clinical medicine and surgery. 2nd edition. St Louis (MO): Saunders; 2004. p. 257–68.

56. Morrissey J, McEntee J. Therapeutic options for thymoma in the rabbit. J Exot Pet Med 2005;14(3):175–81.

57. Guzman D, Mayer J, Gould J, et al. Radiation therapy for the treatment of thymoma in rabbits (Oryctolagus cuniculus). J Exot Pet Med 2006;15(2):138–44, 5.

58. Prélaud AR, Lee AJD, Mueller RS, et al. Presumptive paraneoplastic exfoliative dermatitis in four domestic rabbits. Vet Rec 2013;172:155.

59. Vernau KM, Grahn BH, Clarke-Scott HA, et al. Thymoma in a geriatric rabbit with hypercalcemia and periodic exophthalmos. J Am Vet Med Assoc 1995;206(6): 820–2.

60. Greenacre CB. Spontaneous tumors of small mammals. Vet Clin North Am Exot Anim Pract 2004;7(3):627–51.

61. Field KJ, Griffith JW, Lang CM. Spontaneous reproductive tract leiomyomas in aged guinea pigs. J Comp Pathol 1989;101:287–94.

62. Collins BR. Common diseases and medical management of rodents and lagamorphs. In: Jacobson ER, Kolias GV, editors. Exotic animals. New York: Churchill Livingstone; 1988. p. 261–316.

63. Gibbons P, Garner M. Mammary gland tumors in guinea pigs (Cavia porcellus). Proceedings of the Association of Exotic Mammal Veterinarians. Milwaukee (WI), August 12–15, 2009.

64. Edigar RD, Kovatch RM. Spontaneous tumors in the Dunkin-Harley guinea pig. J Natl Cancer Inst 1976;56:293–4.

65. Woodruff-Pak DS, Trojanowski JQ. The older rabbit as an animal model: implications for Alzheimer's disease. Neurobiol Aging 1996;17(2):283–90.

66. Woodruf-Pak DS, Green JT, Pak JT, et al. The long-term effect of nefiracetam on learning in older rabbits. Behav Brain Res 2002;136:299–308.

67. Bradley Bays T, Lightfoot T, Mayer J. Exotic pet behavior — birds, reptiles, and small mammals. St Louis (MO): Saunders Elsevier; 2006.

68. Thompson L. Recognition and assessment of pain in small exotic mammals. In: Egger CM, Love L, Doherty T, editors. Pain management in veterinary practice. Hoboken (NJ): Wiley; 2013. p. 399–408.

69. Carmel B, Johnson. Euthanasia of exotic pets. In: Proceedings of the Australian Veterinary Association Annual Conference. Perth (Australia), 2008.
70. Clarke GL, Allen AM, Small JD, et al. Subclinical Scurvy in a guinea pig. Vet Pathol 1980;17:40–4.
71. Mitchell MA, Tully TN. Manual of Exotic pet practice. Saint Louis, MO: Elsevier Health Sciences; 2008.
72. Flecknell P, Waterman-Pearson A. Pain management in animals. St Louis (MO): WB Saunders; 2000.
73. Flecknell PA. Analgesia and post-operative care. In: Flecknell P, editor. Laboratory animal anesthesia. 4th ediiton. Boston: Academic Pres; 2016. p. 141–92.
74. Flecknell PA. Analgesia of small mammals. Vet Clin North Am Exot Anim Pract 2001;4(1):47–56. Hernandez-Divers SJ, Lennox AM.
75. Lichtenberger M. Sedation and anesthesia in exotic companion mammals. Association of Avian Veterinarians. Milwaukee (WI), August 12–15, 2009.
76. Ko J. Anesthesia and analgesia for small mammals and birds. Vet Clin North Am Exot Anim Pract 2007;1(10):293–315.
77. Plumb DC. Plumb's veterinary drug handbook. 8th ediiton. Ames (IA): Willey Blackwell Publishing; 2015.
78. Uebelhart D, Thonar EJ, Zhang JW, et al. Protective effect of exogenous chondroitin 4,6-sulfate in the acute degradation of articular cartilage in the rabbit. Osteoarthritis Cartilage 1998;6:6–13.
79. Fisher P, Graham J. Rabbits. In: Carpenter JW, Marion CJ, editors. Exotic animal formulary. 5th editon. St Louis (MO): Elsevier; 2017. p. 494–531.
80. Takihaa K, Azuma J, Awata N, et al. Beneficial effect of taurine in rabbits with chronic congestive heart failure. Am Heart J 1986;112(6):1278–84.
81. Available at: www.lapoflove.com. Accessed July 30, 2019.
82. How to Say Goodbye, Andy Roark, DVM APRIL 16, 2019. Available at: http://www.vetstreet.com/our-pet-experts/dr-andy-roark-bio. Accessed July 30, 2019.

Geriatric Invertebrates

Sarah Pellett, MA, VetMB, CertAVP(ZM), DZooMed(Reptilian), MRCVS[a],*,
Michelle O'Brien, BVetMed, CertZooMed, DECZM(ZHM), MRCVS[b],
Benjamin Kennedy, MSc, BVetMed, MRCVS, Mem RES[c]

KEYWORDS

- Invertebrate • Arthropod • Mollusk • Aging • Disease

KEY POINTS

- Invertebrates may have complex life cycles and several factors may contribute to the timing of the life cycle, such as husbandry factors. The breeding status and gender of the invertebrate may also affect the life span.
- Visual signs may be apparent in aging invertebrates, to include loss of limbs, wing damage, or color changes caused by physical degeneration.
- Deterioration in body condition may be observed as the arthropod ages, with the loss of the tarsi in beetles and Orthoptera (grasshoppers, locusts, crickets, and cockroaches) commonly seen. Color fading may also be observed, and this has been frequently seen in fruit beetles.
- Fluid therapy, orally or parenterally administered, may be necessary in cases where supportive care is required.
- Euthanasia may be an option for arthropods, spiders, and snails with age-related disease and unmanageable conditions.

INTRODUCTION

With advancement in veterinary medicine, pets of all species are living much longer; however, several factors need to be considered when discussing the concept of aging in an invertebrate. Invertebrates may have complex life cycles and husbandry factors may contribute to the speed of the life cycle. Some animals undergo an ultimate (final) molt and some continue to molt throughout their lives. The breeding status and gender of the invertebrate may also affect the life span.

As in any species, older pets may display subtle changes that may go unnoticed until the problem has become more advanced. In contrast with other taxa, invertebrate clients do not often visit the veterinary clinic for regular wellness visits. Invertebrates are increasingly seen in zoologic collections, animal care teaching colleges, schools, and research/scientific laboratories, as pets or study animals. Although invertebrate

[a] Animates Veterinary Clinic, 2 The Green, Thurlby, Lincolnshire PE10 0EB, UK; [b] Wildfowl & Wetlands Trust, Newgrounds Lane, Slimbridge, Gloucestershire GL2 7BT, UK; [c] Anton Vets, Anton Trading Estate, Anton Mill Road, Andover SP10 2NJ, UK
* Corresponding author.
E-mail address: sarah_pellett@hotmail.com

Vet Clin Exot Anim 23 (2020) 595–613
https://doi.org/10.1016/j.cvex.2020.05.002
1094-9194/20/© 2020 Elsevier Inc. All rights reserved.
vetexotic.theclinics.com

medicine is still in its infancy compared with other exotic pet species, there has been more of a demand from both owners and veterinarians seeking advice in treating these animals over the last few years.[1]

The range of invertebrates is vast, ranging from single-celled protozoa to multicellular mollusks, arthropods, worms, leeches, sponges, and corals, but the animals most likely to be pertinent to the general practitioner are members of the Arthropoda (organisms having a hard, jointed exoskeleton and paired, jointed legs) and Mollusca (snails, slugs, mussels, oysters, clams, octopuses, nautiluses, squids, cuttlefish) phyla.[2] Information regarding geriatric invertebrates is sparse in the literature compared with other taxa, and information provided in this article is a combination of scientific publications and personal experience/anecdotal reports gained from several highly experienced keepers and colleagues. This article discusses aging in many invertebrate species but with a focus on species likely to be seen in general practice within the phyla Arthropoda and Mollusca.

INVERTEBRATE LIFE SPAN

Spider keepers can become extremely attached to their pets because of the longevity of females, especially if they have kept and reared them from a small spiderling stage (often <5 mm in leg span) up to adult size (>13 cm in leg span for many species).[3] In some theraphosid (tarantula) species, females may live more than 30 years, with the oldest known individual reported to have lived 42 years.[4,5] In comparison, male spiders generally live for approximately 3 to 4 years, often perishing up to a year following their terminal (ultimate) molt.

Giant African land snails (**Fig. 1**) are also popular as pets and can be presented to the veterinary practitioner for assessment and advice. They have a life span of approximately 5 to 8 years, although some may reach 10 years of age.[6]

Land hermit crabs, *Coenobita clypeatus* and *Coenobita compressus*, are also kept within collections and as pets. They have been reported to live up to 15 years in captivity, with some individuals living to more than 20 years of age.[7] In the wild, ages of up to 30 years have been reported.[8]

Scorpions are sometimes kept as pets, and the most commonly kept species is the North African imperial or emperor scorpion, *Pandinus imperator*, which can live up to 8 years in captivity.[7]

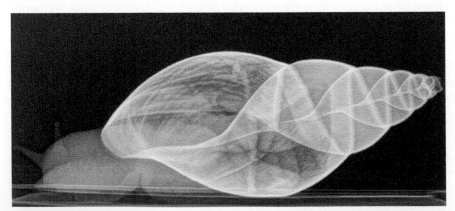

Fig. 1. Radiograph of an adult giant African land snail. (*Courtesy of* R.J. Harvey, BVetMed(-Hons) MRCVS, Keighley, UK.)

FACTORS INFLUENCING LIFE SPAN

As previously stated, the life cycle and therefore the aging process in invertebrates can be highly variable and highly complex. In general, an insect or spider in a position of artificial abundance (typical of a private pet) goes through its life cycle more quickly. Many invertebrates have optimal light cycles, temperatures, and food abundance that are associated with a shorter life span because the life cycle occurs more efficiently. In insect rearing systems, this is a desirable trait because it allows rapid breeding, but this may not be the case in other systems. Nutritional and disease status of the parent insect can also influence the speed at which progeny go through their life cycles. When overall life expectancy is the overall goal, then careful considerations with respect to husbandry and diet are often important. Typically, a modest feed intake alongside carefully controlled temperature and day length are associated with a longer life. This outcome may not be associated with a lower level of welfare but may be a reflection of the natural biology of the species involved.

AGING INVERTEBRATES

In the first instance, invertebrates that have undertaken repeated ecdysis can be aged by size and presence of anatomic features. Often features that are associated with age in older animals can be normal in animals that are actively going through their normal life cycles; for example, phasmids and mantids can sustain damage but this damage may be resolved with the next molt.

Visual features of a geriatric invertebrate can include the loss of limbs, wing damage, color change, and the presence of melanization lesions. Erosions of the distal limbs or on the cuticle, as well as a general lessening in body condition, can also be present. The nature of visual features of aging depends on whether the animal molts throughout its life, undergoes an ultimate molt, or molts at all. In invertebrates that undergo an ultimate molt, lesions associated with general wear and tear are most present, because an animal that undergoes molting throughout its life typically displays more subtle signs, such as a lessening in body condition.

The age of an insect affects many factors of its life, such as behavior, reproductive output, insecticide detoxification and susceptibility, and vectorial capacity (ie, the capacity of an insect to bite a host).[9] To determine the age of an insect, many methods have been described in the scientific literature, but these methods may have limitations, and are often based on a few samples and on a single sex. Methods of aging insects described in the literature include measuring and observing ovarian follicles, counting cuticular bands, assessing and grading the amount of body fat present, and assessing cuticular degradation.[10] Another method to determine the age of an invertebrate is to evaluate pteridine pigments in an individual.[9] Pteridines are purine-based pigment molecules and were first described in 1891 in butterfly wings.[11-13] The age of some species of invertebrates can be calculated by measuring pteridine concentration, which accumulates as the insect ages; however, there are limitations. This method has been reported in the formicine ant, Polyrhachis sexpinosa, but the study showed that only head weight and not pteridine concentration were correlated with the age of the invertebrate.[14] Pteridine concentration to age an invertebrate has been reported in the pink-spotted bollworm, Pectinophora scutigera, in which 6-biopterin was isolated and used to calculate the concentration of pteridines.[15] In that study, 6-biopterin was isolated from pink bollworm moths at different ages but the investigators did not prove a correlation with increasing age.[15] Pteridine concentration to determine age has been studied in some dipteran species and the investigators concluded that other parameters, such as light intensity, sex, and temperature, may affect pteridines with age.[16] In a more recent publication, pteridine levels were shown to increase with age in the honeybee, *Apis mellifera*, although variation in the data generated a 4-day range in age estimation.[9]

Publications on gastropods have described amputations of eyes and tentacles and, in 1 article, the age of the animal was described to affect regeneration.[17] The giant African land snail *Achatina fulica* was used to investigate the ability of regeneration of the eye. The degree of regeneration was deduced by light-microscopic and electrophysiologic methods and by analyzing the motor response to visual stimuli. In older snails, the number of regenerated eye-bearing tentacles decreased, whereas the period of regeneration increased.[17] The investigators reported that aging significantly affected regeneration time from 2 weeks to several weeks and, as far as they were aware, this phenomenon had not been reported in other gastropods.[17]

AGING OF THE INVERTEBRATE IMMUNE SYSTEM

In many species, immunity declines with age, a process that has been referred to as immune senescence, and invertebrates are no exception to this.[18–20] Numerous publications are found within the literature describing significant decreases in antibacterial activity with age, melanization potential, and number of hemocytes (blood corpuscles) in many taxa to include mosquitoes,[21–26] flies,[21,22] dragonflies,[27] scorpionflies,[28] crickets,[29] butterflies,[30,31] and bees.[32–34] In some species, because of immune senescence, a decrease in immunity in aging invertebrates is associated with a higher predisposition to parasite burdens.[24,35] However, in many of these studies with conclusions suggesting that older invertebrates are more susceptible to higher parasite burdens because of a weakened immune system, there has not been a definitive assessment of immune function and parasite susceptibility.[18] Other studies have challenged the theory that older invertebrates are more prone to infection and have shown that older insects are more resistant to a range of pathogens. Older mosquitoes have been shown to be significantly more resistant to plasmodium infection than younger conspecifics; however, the age effect is reversed when older mosquitoes have taken 1 previous noninfected blood meal.[18] The authors have concluded that structural and functional alterations in the invertebrates' physiology with age may be more crucial than immunity in determining the probability of plasmodium infection in elderly mosquitoes.

INVERTEBRATE ONCOLOGY

Neoplasia in invertebrates has been reported in the literature across many invertebrate taxa and is more commonly documented in mollusks and insects and less frequently in Cnidaria (any invertebrate animal, such as a hydra, jellyfish, sea anemone, or coral, considered as belonging to the phylum Cnidaria, characterized by the specialized stinging structures in the tentacles surrounding the mouth; a coelenterate), crustaceans, and spiders.[36] Neoplasia is yet to be reported in Porifera (the phylum of sponges) and Echinodermata (the phylum including starfishes and sea urchins)[37] Genetic alterations to invertebrate cells can be spontaneous, hereditary, or acquired, and consequentially results in proliferation caused by lack of response of the normal regulatory cell growth controls.[38,39] In several reports on invertebrate neoplasia, the cause has been reported to be unknown, but, as more invertebrates are kept in collections, aging must be a consideration, although scientific studies are required to support this. Reports of neoplasia in the butter clam, *Saxidomus giganteus*, have suggested that environmental contaminants may be a factor, but others have described the causes of neoplasia to be spontaneous.[40,41]

Suspected neoplasia can be a cause of a veterinary visit, because clients often mistake abscesses, retained cuticle, or cuticular degeneration for neoplasia. Genuine neoplasia is considered by the authors to be a rare finding.

NEMATODES

Caenorhabditis elegans, a powerful soil-dwelling nematode model for analysis of the conserved mechanisms that modulate healthy aging, has been used in numerous studies related to factors that accelerate or slow the aging process.[42] Both wild-type and laboratory-adapted strains have been used in research. Mitochondrially defective mutants live longer than wild-type animals, and loss-of-function mutations in clk-1 increase life span, as also occurs in mice.[43,44]

An insulin/insulinlike growth factor I–like signaling pathway determines the rate of aging of the adult nematode, and mutations in genes encoding this pathway can result in a doubling of life span. Despite long-lived mutants appearing healthy, they show a heavy fitness cost consistent with an evolutionary theory of aging.[45] Interestingly, mutations affecting the age-1 gene, which slows aging of the animal, result in significant delays in the development of sarcopenia.[46]

Exposure to environmental stressors, such as caloric restriction or exposure to mild stress, can increase stress resistance and life span in *C elegans*.[47]

Several natural substances have also been found to slow the process of aging in this nematode, including *Ganoderma lucidum*, a fungus that regulates the biophysiologic processes in the nematodes through multiple signaling pathways, and *Ribes fasciculatum*, a deciduous shrub that confers increased longevity and stress resistance.[48,49]

Several drugs (including some antioxidants), metabolites, and synthetic compounds have also been found to effectively increase the longevity or delay the aging of nematodes and insects. These substances include 2-bromo-4'-nitroacetophenone,[50] catalpol,[51] astragalan,[52] L-theanine,[53] wheat gluten hydrolysate,[54] glaucarubinone,[55] lonidamine,[56] and resveratrol.[57]

In 1 study, the rate at which wild-type *C elegans* was killed by bacterial pathogens increased as nematodes aged.[58] However, there is some evidence that supports that older invertebrates can be less susceptible to infection, possibly through having been exposed to more pathogens over their life spans, so that they have some immunologic memory to withstand an infection. It is also possible that, because of epigenetic effects and changes in the ability to express genes required by an infecting/infectious pathogen, age in a host invertebrate could bring about an advantage. Anecdotally, this is seen in a tropical freshwater snail *Biomphalaria glabrata*, a secondary obligate host for the water-borne parasitic human disease schistosomiasis or bilharzia. Older snails are harder to infect with the flesh-burrowing parasite and this is thought to be caused by the snail's inability to relocate a gene, advantageous to the parasite, to an active area of the cell nucleus for upregulation of gene expression.[59]

CNIDARIA

Jellyfish (class: Scyphozoa) have complex life cycles, with the medusae of most species being dioecious (denoting species in which male and female genitals do not occur in the same individual).[60] The fertilized egg develops into a planula (ciliated, free-swimming larva). The planktonic larvae settle to the bottom and then develop into sessile polyps with tentacles. At this stage, the animal can reproduce asexually, by budding or formation of podocysts.[60] Under the correct conditions, strobilation occurs, where segmentation and metamorphosis occur, and the segmented parts of the polyp become incipient medusae. These medusae then become free-swimming ephyrae (larvae) and the life cycle is then completed by growing into adult medusae.[60] They only live as medusae for approximately 1 year, but the polyps can live up to 25 years (D. Clarke, Zoological Society of London, personal communication, 2019).

Turritopsis nutricula belongs to the class Hydrozoa and has been extensively studied because of its ability to undergo ontogeny reversal at all stages of medusa growth, including the adult stage with mature gonads.[61] The potential for reverse development could be present, but hidden, in other cnidarians.[62] Within Anthozoa, only coral primary polyps can revert to planula larvae, but available information on Staurozoa and Cubozoa is scant and the life cycles of many cnidarians still need to be determined, so it is likely that other cases of reverse development exist.[62]

COMMON SIGNS ASSOCIATED WITH AGING OBSERVED ACROSS TAXA
Theraphosids (Tarantula Spiders)

The opisthosoma (equivalent to the abdomen) can decrease in anorexic animals, adult males, and sometimes in elderly specimens (**Fig. 2**). Similar to insects, ultimate molt males often accumulate damage and the associated melanization as they age. There have also been reports of increased incidents of problems during ecdysis (S. Baker, Venomtech, personal communication, 2019).

Anecdotally, venom yield may decrease as the theraphosid ages (S. Trim and S. Baker, Venomtech, personal communication). Older spiders seem less able to climb on smooth surfaces (S. Baker, Venomtech, personal communication, 2019).

Other Arachnids

Poor web building has been noted in aging orb spiders, which consequentially leads to lack of food (D. Clarke, Zoological Society of London, personal communication, 2019). This problem has also been noted in older theraphosid spiders (S. Baker, Venomtech, personal communication, 2019).

Gastropods (Snails)

It is common to be presented with an elderly snail with the mantle having separated from the rest of the body (**Fig. 3**). Often there are other underlying issues to consider

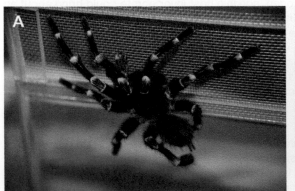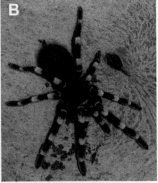

Fig. 2. (*A*) Aging theraphosid with an opisthosoma decreased in size. (*B*) Young theraphosid (*Acanthoscurria* spp) with a normal-sized opisthosoma for comparison purposes. ([A] *Courtesy of* Hummingbird Studios, Lincolnshire, UK.)

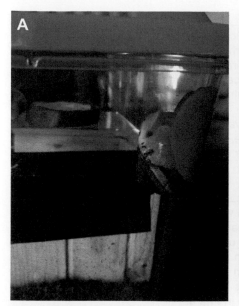
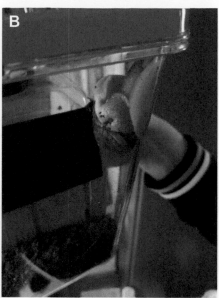

Fig. 3. (*A, B*) Demonstrate mantle separation in a garden snail (*Cornu aspersum*). (*Courtesy of* D. Franchi, Prato, Italy.)

and a grave prognosis must be given, but if the snail is placed in a shallow tank to restrict climbing, then this occasionally repairs.[6]

In aging snails, there may be wearing of the periostracum, the thin outermost layer of the shell in gastropods, and this has been reported to be very noticeable in old *Partula* shells where the markings fade away (D. Clarke, Zoological Society of London, personal communication, 2019). *Partula* snails were once common on islands in French Polynesia but suffered huge population declines, in most part caused by predation by an introduced carnivorous snail in a failed attempt at biological control. Many zoologic collections are involved in captive breeding of several *Partula* species for eventual reintroduction to the wild.

Snails may present with prolapse of organs (often the digestive tract) through their mouthparts (**Fig. 4**). Digestive tract prolapses usually occur in chronically unwell or geriatric snails and often indicate severe systemic disease. Euthanasia is usually advised on welfare grounds.

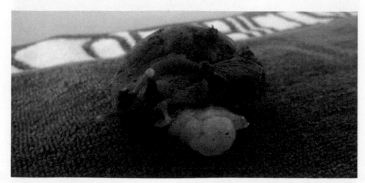

Fig. 4. Prolapse of digestive tract through mouthparts of an African land snail.

Lepidoptera (Butterflies and Moths)

Aging Lepidoptera may present with significant wing damage and loss of scales and/or loss of coloration (Clarke, personal communication, 2019) **(Fig. 5)**. If the butterfly or moth with a section of wing missing is required to continue breeding, there is an option to repair the wing using a wing from a deceased butterfly or a cardboard splint. For detailed information on exoskeleton repair please refer to relevant publications in the literature.[63]

In the wild, Lepidoptera can have highly variable life spans depending on the season and their migratory behavior. For example, the well-known monarch butterfly has a short life span (5–8 weeks) in the summer months but has a significantly longer life span (up to 9 months) when migrating.

Mantodea (Mantids)

Mantids all undergo an ultimate molt from which they typically breed. When actively molting, many invertebrates, including mantids, can molt cuticular damage away, but are unable to do this once within the ultimate molt. Geriatric mantids can have black melanization lesions associated with the general wear and tear that occurs as they live. These lesions can be present on the eyes, limbs, and occasionally on the abdomen. Erosion can occur on the ends of the limbs, and eventually entire limbs can be lost. Examples of this can be seen in **Fig. 6**.

Older mantids can get a so-called black-eye syndrome, which is associated with melanization of the eyes and limbs. There are some preliminary data that suggest that ovarian degeneration can occur in female mantids that are unbred and that this may result in an overall shorter life expectancy. This condition may be associated with an increased bacterial or fungal load. Supportive treatment with oral fluids seems to reduce severity of clinical signs.

Other Arthropods

A decline in body condition may be seen as the arthropod ages, with the loss of the tarsi in beetles and Orthoptera commonly seen (D. Clarke, Zoological Society of London, personal communication, 2019). Limb loss in phasmids is also commonly seen

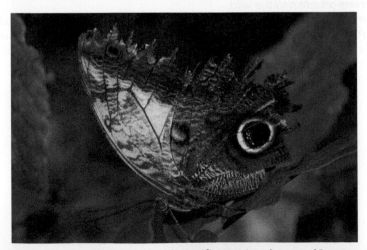

Fig. 5. Aging Lepidoptera (*Caligo* spp) with significant wing damage. (*Courtesy of* S. Hall, Slimbridge, UK.)

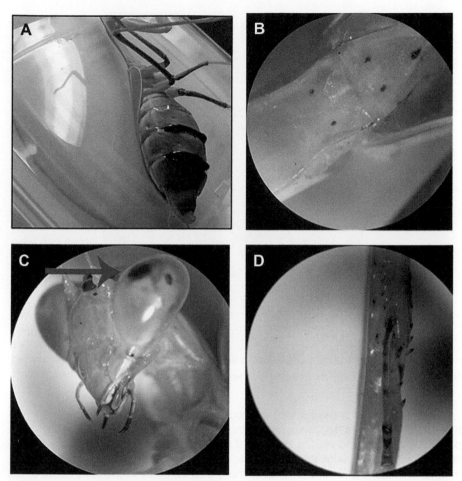

Fig. 6. Features present on an aging mantis. Melanization occurs secondary to the general wear and tear on the cuticle. (*A*) The ventral membranes that can extrude between the segments. (*B*) Surface melanization lesions in an elderly female mantis. (*C*) Black-eye melanization lesion in an elderly male mantis (*arrow*). (*D*) Typical melanization present on forelimbs.

(**Fig. 7**). Color fading may also be observed, and this has frequently been seen in fruit beetles (D. Clarke, Zoological Society of London, personal communication, 2019). Pigmentation changes can also be seen in other invertebrates, such as the glassy-winged sharpshooter, *Homalodisca vitripennis*. Over the duration of its life span, a red pigment contained in the wing veins darkens and becomes black/brown.[64] Anecdotally, it has been suggested that lighter colored scorpions take on a more opaque appearance as they get older. This change has not been observed in darker scorpions, but this may possibly be because of the color obscuring opacification (S. Baker, Venomtech, personal communication, 2019).

The loss of fertility has been anecdotally reported in several species; for example, jewel wasp females (D. Clarke, Zoological Society of London, personal communication, 2019). Anecdotally it has been reported that there is a loss of control by pheromones in Hymenoptera (eg, honeybees and leaf-cutter ants) as the animal ages (D. Clarke, Zoological Society of London, personal communication, 2019).

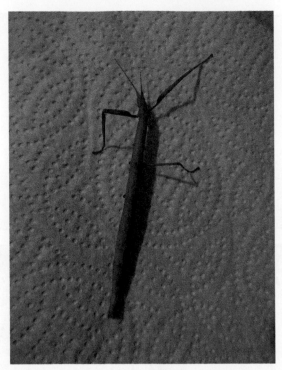

Fig. 7. Limb loss in an elderly Indian stick insect (*Carausius morosus*).

In arthropods that live in colonies or groups, it is important to know the age structure. In some species (eg, myriapods; arthropods of a group that includes the centipedes, millipedes, and related animals), if 1 dies and is not quickly removed it can lead to a release of toxins that can lead to mortality in other members of the group. In other species (eg, ants), the death of the queen can lead to the slow death of the entire colony.

Cnidaria

Jellyfish can deteriorate generally with old age, and observations include a deterioration in normal body structure when geriatric, especially loss of oral arms (D. Clarke, Zoological Society of London, personal communication).

MANAGEMENT OF AGING INVERTEBRATES

In contrast with other taxa, where there are multimodal approaches to treating and managing geriatric patients, there is limited information and availability to treat the aging invertebrate. Invertebrates are often not given the same ethical consideration; however, with the number of invertebrates being kept and clients seeking advice, clinicians have a duty of care to provide optimal care.

Clinicians must view each case on an individual basis and consider the welfare of the animal, taking into consideration possible adaptations to the environment and husbandry. Management change is an essential component to managing the clinical signs of aging in invertebrates. As invertebrates age, their ability to navigate around their enclosures can become reduced, especially if they have lost limbs. Introducing further climbing areas, rough surfaces, or perching points can be helpful in allowing normal behavior. In addition to this, reducing the vertical space within an enclosure can reduce the damage that may occur should the invertebrate fall. This measure is especially important to elderly snails and new world theraphosid spiders. Invertebrates that may be cannibalized within a population may be more appropriately managed alone or within a geriatric group (eg, African land snails within a group).

Ensuring that food is provided within easy reach for aged invertebrates that may have lost limbs and therefore have reduced climbing ability is also an important consideration for their welfare. The potential of the animal feeling pain must also be considered. It has not been proved whether invertebrates experience pain or are simply showing a reflexive response to a painful stimulus.[65] There are nerve endings or similar sensory structures within internal tissues and the body wall present in arthropods and mollusks. In cephalopods, there are well-developed nervous systems and brains together with demonstration of complex behaviors, including the ability to respond to environmental cues.[66–68] Many invertebrate species have endogenous opioids and respond to noxious stimuli, and some species also respond to exogenous opioids.[69–77] The paucity of publications accentuates the need for further research on analgesia use in invertebrates, but analgesia doses (although most are anecdotal) may be found in exotic animal formularies and publications. In 1 study, administration of morphine at 50 to 100 mg/kg intracelomically, or administration of butorphanol at 20 mg/kg, was shown to decrease responses to noxious stimuli in theraphosids.[78] Hypothermia is not considered a humane method of anesthesia or analgesia because there is no loss of sensation. In many arthropods, an increased plane of nutrition following the final molt can result in the animal moving through its life cycle at a rapid pace, therefore reducing the feed of such animals can be helpful for extending life span and the associated morbidity.

Fluid therapy administered orally or parenterally may be required in cases where supportive care is required (**Figs. 8** and **9**).[63] In some cases, where age-related damage is associated with a bacterial infection, antibiotics may play a role in improving clinical signs.

A detailed account of diagnostic techniques for invertebrates is beyond the scope of this article, but these are summarized later to give guidance on approaches that can be used to determine a diagnosis in these animals.

Hemolymph may be aspirated from invertebrates; the authors prefer to take hemolymph from tarantulas with the animal under inhalable anesthesia (eg, with isoflurane). The sample is collected from the heart with needle placement (30-gauge insulin needle and syringe) in the dorsal midline of the opisthosoma. Pressure is applied to the site of needle insertion and this often achieves hemostasis, but a small amount of tissue adhesive may also be applied to the cuticle. Two recent studies have assessed plasma biochemistry of hemolymph in Chilean rose tarantulas and readers are encouraged to refer to these recent publications for more details.[79,80] In snails, methods have been described where hemolymph has been collected by drilling into the shell and aspirating a sample from the heart or by incising the mantle and then into the visceral sac.[81–83] A less invasive method preferred by the authors is to locate the pneumostome (the respiratory opening; **Fig. 10**) and collect hemolymph ventral to this. For *Achatina* spp weighing less than 50 g, the insertion site is approximately 5 mm ventral to the pneumostome. For snails weighing 200 g, the insertion point is approximately 20 mm ventral to the pneumostome.[84]

Cytology may provide evidence of the presence of bacterial, fungal, and protozoal causative agents from the skin surface, oral or anal discharges, and feces. Fecal analysis may be valuable to identify protozoans and gregarines. Skin scrapings must be performed with care to avoid penetration of the delicate exoskeleton.

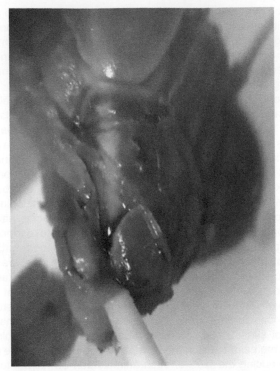

Fig. 8. Stereomicroscopy of placement of catheter end to provide oral critical care solution to a mantid.

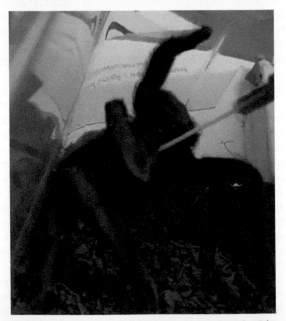

Fig. 9. Oral administration of critical care solution in theraphosid spider.

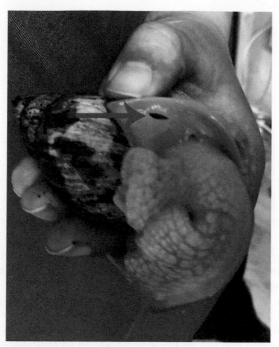

Fig. 10. The respiratory opening (*arrow*) in a giant African land snail. (*Courtesy of* A. Plant, Lincolnshire, UK.)

Sampling of secretions with a charcoal swab for bacterial and fungal culture and sensitivity can be performed, especially if cytology is supportive of an infection. Interpretation of results must be taken with caution because pathogens are often difficult to culture using the standard technique, commensal microbial populations are not described in the literature, and culture temperatures may need to be decreased as a result of the poikilothermic nature of most invertebrates.[85]

Euthanasia

Except for cephalopods, in the United Kingdom, invertebrates are not governed by the same legislation and standards as are vertebrate species. Further information on euthanasia for invertebrate taxa can be found in documents specifically produced to outline ethical and humane euthanasia techniques.[86,87] Euthanasia must be taken into consideration for invertebrates with age-related disease and unmanageable conditions.

Adequate analgesia and/or anesthesia must be provided before euthanasia. In general, this can be provided via inhalable anesthesia, although there are some exceptions; for example, the giant African land snail, which is better anesthetized through transmucosal or injectable anesthesia. Hypothermia is not deemed a humane method of anesthesia or analgesia because there is no loss of sensation, and it is strongly discouraged. Once anesthetized, pentobarbitone can be injected into the hemocelom (the body cavity that contains hemolymph).[88] Death can be confirmed by the cessation of heart rate with a Doppler probe. Gaseous anesthesia is not endorsed for terrestrial snails because of the potential of causing stress, because excess mucus production has been reported with this method.[86] The recommended protocol to euthanize a giant African land snail is by using a bath of 100% phenoxyethanol (Aqua-Sed, VETARK Professional) to cover the

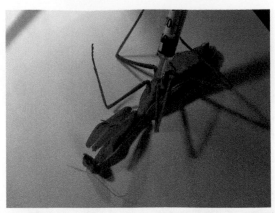

Fig. 11. Site for euthanizing via central ganglion in an anesthetized mantid.

muscular foot. Sodium pentobarbitone can be administered into the body cavity (personal communication, R. Saunders, 2013) once unresponsive and cessation of a heartbeat confirmed using an 8-MHz Doppler probe.[89]

Other methods of euthanasia published involve administration of potassium chloride, resulting in hyperkalosis. In theraphosids, this is administered into the prosoma ganglia via the sternum or into the heart.[90] In other species, such as phasmids, the injection is administered into the ventral midline, at the junction between the first leg plate and adjacent ventral plate. This method has also been extrapolated for Mantidae (**Fig. 11**).[90]

SUMMARY

Invertebrates are becoming more popular within the pet trade and among teaching colleges, schools, and zoologic collections. As collections age, clients may seek veterinary intervention where the welfare of the animal must be considered. Supportive care may be an option, but euthanasia must be considered for invertebrates with age-related unmanageable conditions.

ACKNOWLEDGMENTS

The authors would like to thank colleagues and organizations that have contributed in expanding invertebrate knowledge; colleagues at the British and Irish Association of Zoos and Aquariums (BIAZA) Terrestrial Invertebrate Working Group for their continued work on increasing awareness of invertebrate husbandry and welfare; and members of the Veterinary Invertebrate Society, an international association of veterinarians, veterinary nurses, scientists, and keepers interested in, and working with, invertebrates. The authors would like to thank Dave Clarke, Steven Trim, and Stuart Baker for sharing their knowledge on aging invertebrates from their collections. The authors are grateful to Professor John Cooper and Mrs Margaret Cooper for their ongoing support and advice on the subject. The authors would like to acknowledge the Royal College of Veterinary Surgeons (RCVS) library for performing a literature review on this topic.

DISCLOSURE

The authors have nothing to disclose.

REFERENCES

1. Pellett S, Kubiak M. A review of invertebrate cases seen in practice. Proceedings Veterinary Invertebrate Society Summer Scientific Meeting. 12th July, 2017. Cambridge, UK: 4.
2. Cooper JE. Skin disease in invertebrates. In: Locke PH, Harvey RG, Mason IS, editors. Manual of small animal dermatology. Cheltenham (UK): British Small Animal Veterinary Association (BSAVA); 1993. p. 198–212.
3. Marnell C. Tarantula and hermit crab emergency care. Vet Clin North Am Exot Anim Pract 2016;19:627–46.
4. Bennie NAC, Loaring CD, Trim SA. Laboratory husbandry of arboreal tarantulas (Theraphosidae) and evaluation of environmental enrichment. Anim Technol 2011;10:163–9.
5. Mason LD, Wardell-Johnson G, Main BY. The longest-lived spider: mygalomorphs dig deep and persevere. Pac Conserv Biol 2018;24:203.
6. O'Brien M. Dealing with giant African land snails. Veterinary Times 2009; 39(18):36–7.
7. Pizzi R. Invertebrates. In: Meredith A, Johnson-Delaney CA, editors. BSAVA manual of exotic pets. 5th edition. Gloucester (UK): BSAVA Publications; 2010. p. 373–85.
8. Smith SA, Scimeca JM, Mainous ME. Culture and maintenance of selected invertebrates in the laboratory and classroom. ILAR J 2011;52:153–64.
9. Rinkevich FD, Margitta JW, Pittman JM, et al. Pteridine levels and head weights are correlated with age and colony task in the honey bee, Apis mellifera. Peer J 2016;4:e2155.
10. Hayes EJ, Wall R. Age-grading adult insects: a review of techniques. Physiol Entomol 1999;24:1–10.
11. Wigglesworth VB. The life of insects. Minneapolis (MN): Weidenfeld and Nicolson; 1964.
12. Zeigler I, Harmsen R. The biology of pteridines in insects. Adv Insect Physiol 1969;6:139–203.
13. Hopkins FG. Pigments in yellow butterflies. Nature 1891;45:197–8.
14. Robson SKA, Crozier RH. An evaluation of two biochemical methods of age determination in insects (pteridines and lipfuscin) using the ant Polyrachis sexpinosa Latrielle (Hymenoptera: Formicidae). Aust J Entomol 2009;48:102–6.
15. Noble RM, Walker PW. Pteridine compounds in adults of the pink spotted bollworm, Pectinophora scutigera. Entomol Exp Appl 1990;57:77–83.
16. Robson SKA, Vickers M, Blows MW, et al. Age determination in individual wild-caught Drosophila serrata using pteridine concentration. J Exp Biol 2006;209: 3155–63.
17. Tartakovskaya OS, Borisenko SL, Zhukov VV. Role of the age factor in eye regeneration in the gastropod Achatina fulica. Biol Bull Acad Sci USSR 2003;30(3): 228–35.
18. Pigeault R, Nicot A, Gandon S, et al. Mosquito age and avian malaria infection. Malar J 2015;14:383.
19. Rodrigues J, Brayner FA, Alves LC, et al. Hemocyte differentiation mediates innate memory in Anopheles gambiae mosquitoes. Science 2010;329:1353–5.
20. Bell G. Evolutionary and nonevolutionary theories of senescence. Am Nat 1984; 124:600–3.
21. Li J, Tracy JW, Christensen BM. Relationship of hemolymph phenoloxidase and mosquito age in Aedes aegyptii. J Invertebr Pathol 1992;60:188–91.

22. Chun J, Riehle M, Paskewitz SM. Effect of mosquito age and reproductive status on melanization of sephadex beads in *Plasmodium*-refractory and -susceptible strains of *Anopheles gambiae*. J Invertebr Pathol 1995;66:11–7.

23. Schwartz A, Koella JC. Melanization of *Plasmodium falciparum* and C-25 sephadex beads by field-caught *Anopheles gambiae* (Diptera: Culicidae) from southern Tanzania. J Med Entomol 2002;39:84–8.

24. Hillyer JF, Schmidt SL, Fuchs JF, et al. Age-associated mortality in immune challenged mosquitoes (*Aedes aegyptii*) correlates with a decrease in haemocyte numbers. Cell Microbiol 2005;7:39–51.

25. Castillo JC, Robertson AE, Strand MR. Characterization of hemocytes from the mosquitoes *Anopheles gambiae* and *Aedes aegypti*. Insect Biochem Mol Biol 2006;36:891–903.

26. Cornet S, Gandon S, Rivero A. Patterns of phenoloxidase activity in insecticide resistant and susceptible mosquitoes differ between laboratory-selected and wild-caught individuals. Parasit Vectors 2013;6:315.

27. Rolff J. Effects of age and gender on immune function of dragonflies (Odonata, Lestidae) from a wild population. Can J Zool 2001;79:2176–80.

28. Kurtz J. Phagocytosis by invertebrate hemocytes: Causes of individual variation in *Panorpa vulgaris* scorpionflies. Microsc Res Tech 2002;57:456–68.

29. Adamo SA, Jensen M, Younger M. Changes in lifetime immunocompetence in male and female *Gryllus texensis* (formerly *G. integer*): trade-offs between immunity and reproduction. Anim Behav 2001;62:417–25.

30. Stoehr AM. Inter- and intra-sexual variation in immune defence in the cabbage white butterfly (*Pieris rapae L.*) (Lepidoptera: Pieridae) J. Ecol Entomol 2007;32:188–93.

31. Prasai K, Karlsson B. Variation in immune defence in relation to age to age in the green-veined white butterfly (*Pieris napi L.*). J Invertebr Pathol 2012;111:252–4.

32. Doums C, Moret Y, Benelli E, et al. Senescence of immune defence in *Bombus* workers. Ecol Entomol 2002;27:138–44.

33. Wilson-Rich N, Dres ST, Starks PT. The ontogeny of immunity: development of innate immune strength in the honey bee (*Apis mellifera*). J Insect Physiol 2008;54:1392–9.

34. Moret Y, Schmid-Hempel P. Immune responses of bumblebee workers as a function of individual and colony age: senescence versus plastic adjustment of the immune function. Oikos 2009;118:371–8.

35. Roberts KE, Hughes WOH. Immunosenescence and resistance to parasite infection in the honey bee, *Apis mellifera*. J Invertebr Pathol 2014;121:1–6.

36. Peters EC, Smolowitz RM, Reynolds TL. Neoplasia. In: Lewbart GA, editor. Invertebrate medicine. 2nd edition. Chichester (England): John Wiley; 2012. p. 448–525.

37. Newton AL, Lewbart GA. Invertebrate oncology. Vet Clin North Am Exot Anim Pract 2017;20:1–19.

38. Kumar V, Abbas AK, Aster AC. Neoplasia. In: Kumar V, Abbas AK, Aster AC, editors. Robbins and Cotran, pathological basis of disease. 9th edition. Philadelphia: Elsevier; 2015. p. 265–340.

39. Robert J. Comparative study of tumorigenesis and tumor immunity in invertebrates and non-mammalian vertebrates. Dev Comp Immunol 2010;34(9):915–25.

40. Pauley GB. A butter clam (*Saxidomus giganteus*) with a polypoid tumor of the foot. J Invertebr Pathol 1967;9(4):577–9.

41. Odintsova NA, Usheva LN, Yakovlev KV, et al. Naturally occurring and artificially induced tumor-like formations in invertebrates: a search for permanent cell lines. J Exp Mar Bio Ecol 2011;407:241–9.

42. Toth ML, Melentijevic I, Shah LN, et al. Neurite sprouting and synapse deterioration in the aging Caenorhabditis elegans nervous system. J Neurosci 2012; 32(26):8778–90.

43. Ventura N, Rea SL, Testi R. Long-lived C. elegans mitochondrial mutants as a model for human mitochondrial-associated diseases. (Special issue: The nematode Caenorhabditis elegans in aging research). Exp Gerontol 2006;41(10): 974–91.

44. Stepanyan Z, Hughes B, Cliche DO, et al. Genetic and molecular characterization of CLK-1/mCLK1, a conserved determinant of the rate of aging. (Special issue: The nematode Caenorhabditis elegans in aging research). Exp Gerontol 2006; 41(10):940–51.

45. Jenkins NL, McColl G, Lithgow GJ. Fitness cost of extended lifespan in Caenorhabditis elegans. Proc Biol Sci 2004;271(1556):2523–6.

46. Fisher AL. Of worms and women: sarcopenia and its role in disability and mortality. J Am Geriatr Soc 2004;52(7):1185–90.

47. Henderson ST, Johnson TE. daf-16 Integrates developmental and environmental inputs to mediate aging in the nematode Caenorhabditis elegans. Curr Biol 2001; 11(24):1975–80.

48. Cuong VT, WeiDong C, JiaHao S, et al. The anti-oxidation and anti-aging effects of Ganoderma lucidum in Caenorhabditis elegans. Exp Gerontol 2019;117: 99–105.

49. Hoon J, DongSeok C. Anti-aging properties of Ribes fasciculatum in Caenorhabditis elegans. Chin J Nat Med 2016;14(5):335–42.

50. Hui L, MengMeng G, Ting X, et al. Screening lifespan-extending drugs in Caenorhabditis elegans via label propagation on drug-protein networks. BMC Syst Biol 2016;10(Suppl. 4):131.

51. HyunWon S, SeMyung C, MyonHee L, et al. Catalpol modulates lifespan via DAF-16/FOXO and SKN-1/Nrf2 activation in Caenorhabditis elegans. Evidence-based complementary and alternative medicine :article ID 524878. New York: Hindawi Publishing Corporation; 2015.

52. HanRui Z, Ni P, SiQin X, et al. Inhibition of polyglutamine-mediated proteotoxicity by Astragalus membranaceus polysaccharide through the DAF-16/FOXO transcription factor in Caenorhabditis elegans. Biochem J 2012;441(1):417–24.

53. Zarse K, Jabin S, Ristow M. L-theanine extends lifespan of adult Caenorhabditis elegans. Eur J Nutr 2012;51(6):765–8.

54. WeiMing Z, Ting L, Min L, et al. Beneficial effects of wheat gluten hydrolysate to extend lifespan and induce stress resistance in nematode Caenorhabditis elegans. PLoS One 2013;8(9):e74553.

55. Zarse K, Bossecker A, Muller-Kuhrt L, et al. The phytochemical glaucarubinone promotes mitochondrial metabolism, reduces body fat, and extends lifespan of Caenorhabditis elegans. Horm Metab Res 2011;43(4):241–3.

56. Schmeisser S, Zarse K, Ristow M. Lonidamine extends lifespan of adult Caenorhabditis elegans by increasing the formation of mitochondrial reactive oxygen species. Horm Metab Res 2011;43(10):687–92.

57. Zarse K, Schmeisser S, Birringer M, et al. Differential effects of resveratrol and SRT1720 on lifespan of adult Caenorhabditis elegans. Horm Metab Res 2010; 42(12):837–9.

58. Laws TR, Harding SV, Smith MP, et al. Age influences resistance of Caenorhab-ditis elegans to killing by pathogenic bacteria. FEMS Microbiol Lett 2004; 234(2):281–7.
59. Bridger JM, Brindley PJ, Knight M. The snail Biomphalaria glabrata as a model to interrogate the molecular basis of complex human diseases. PLoS Negl Trop Dis 2018;12(8):e0006552.
60. Stoskopf MK. Coelenterates. In: Lewbart GA, editor. Invertebrate medicine. 2nd edition. Chichester (England): John Wiley; 2012. p. 21–56.
61. Piraino S, Boero F, Aeschbach B, et al. Reversing the Life Cycle: Medusae Trans-forming into Polyps and Cell Transdifferentiation in *Turritopsis nutricula* (Cnidaria, Hydrozoa). Biol Bull 1996;190:302–12.
62. Piraino S, DeVito D, Schmich J, et al. Reverse development in Cnidaria. Can J Zool 2004;82:1748–54.
63. Pellett S, O'Brien M. Exoskeleton repair in invertebrates. Vet Clin North Am Exot Anim Pract 2019;22:315–30.
64. Timmons C, Hassell A, Lauziere I, et al. Age determination of the glassy-winged grasshopper, *Homalodisca vitripennis*, using wing pigmentation. J Insect Sci 2011;11:78.
65. Murray MJ. Euthanasia. In: Lewbart GA, editor. Invertebrate medicine. Oxford (England): Blackwell Publishing; 2012. p. 441–3.
66. Cooper JE. Emergency care of invertebrates. Vet Clin North Am Exot Anim Pract 1998;1(1):251–64.
67. Tarsitano MS, Jackson RR. Araneophagic jumping spiders discriminate between detour routes that do and do not lead to prey. Anim Behav 1997;53:257–66.
68. Jackson RR, Carter CM, Tarsitano MS. Trial-and-error solving of a confinement problem by a jumping spider, Portia Fibriata. Behaviour 2001;138:1215–34.
69. Dyakonova VE. Role of opioid peptides in behaviour of invertebrates. J Evol Bio-chem Physiol 2001;37:335–47.
70. Kavaliers M, Hirst M, Teskey GC. A functional role for an opiate system in snail thermal behaviour. Science 1983;220:99–101.
71. Mather JA. Animal suffering: an invertebrate perspective. J Appl Anim Welf Sci 2001;4:151–6.
72. Manev H, Dimitrijevic N. Fruit flies for anti-pain drug discovery. Life Sci 2005;76: 2403–7.
73. Elwood RW, Appel M. Pain experience in hermit crabs? Anim Behav 2009;77: 1243–6.
74. Nathaniela TI, Pankseppb J, Hubera R. Effects of a single and repeated morphine treatment on conditioned and unconditioned behavioral sensitization in Crayfish. Behav Brain Res 2010;207:310–20.
75. Cooper JE. Anesthesia, analgesia, and euthanasia of invertebrates. ILAR J 2011; 52:196–204.
76. Keller DL, Abbott AD, Sladky KK. Invertebrate antinociception: Are opioids effec-tive in tarantulas? Proc Am Assoc Zoo Vet 2012;2012:97.
77. Lewbart GA. Clinical anesthesia and analgesia in invertebrates. J Exot Pet Med 2012;21:59–70.
78. Sladky KK. Current understanding of fish and invertebrate anesthesia and anal-gesia. Proceedings Association of Reptilian and Amphibian Veterinarians. 18th-24th October, 2014. Orlando (FL): p. 122–4.
79. Eichelmann MA, Lewbart GA. Hemolymph chemistry reference ranges of the Chilean Rose tarantula *Grammostola rosea* (Walkenaer, 1837) using the Vetscan

biochemistry analyser based on IFCC-CLSI C28-A$_3$. J Zoo Wildl Med 2018;49(3): 528–34.

80. Kennedy B, Warner A, Trim S. Reference intervals for plasma biochemistry of hemolymph in the Chilean Rose tarantula (*Grammostola rosea*) under chemical restraint. J Zoo Wildl Med 2019;50(1):127–36.

81. Friedl FE. Studies on larval Fascioloides magna. IV Chromatographic analyses of free amino acids in the haemolymph of a host snail. J Parasitol 1961;47:773–6.

82. Williams D. Sample taking in invertebrate veterinary medicine. Vet Clin North Am Exot Anim Pract 1999;2(3):777–801.

83. Brockelman CR. Inhibition of Rhabditis maupasi (Rhabditidae: nematoda), maturation and reproduction by factors from the snail host, Helix aspersa. J Invertebr Pathol 1975;25:229–37.

84. Cooper JE. Bleeding of pulmonate snails. Lab Anim 1994;28:277–8.

85. Braun ME, Heatley JJ, Chitty J. Clinical techniques of invertebrates. Vet Clin North Am Exot Anim Pract 2006;9:205–21.

86. Pellett S, Kubiak M, Pizzi R, et al. BIAZA recommendations for ethical euthanasia of invertebrates. (Version 3.0 - april 2017). 2017. Available at: http://www.biaza. org.uk/In press.

87. Eichelmann M. EAZA Guidelines for the Euthanasia of Invertebrates. Available at: https://www.eaza.net/about-us/eazadocuments/In review.

88. Dombrowski D, De Voe R. Emergency care of Invertebrates. Vet Clin North Am Exot Anim Pract 2007;10(2):621–45.

89. Rees Davies R, Chitty JR, Saunders R. Cardiovascular monitoring of an Achatina snail using a Doppler ultrasound unit. Proceedings of the British Veterinary Zoological Society Autumn Meeting. 2000. RVC. London: 101.

90. Bennie NAC, Loaring CD, Bennie MMG, et al. An effective method for terrestrial arthropod euthanasia. J Exp Biol 2012;215:4237–41.

Geriatric Hedgehogs

Dan H. Johnson, DVM, DABVP (Exotic Companion Mammal)

KEYWORDS

- *Atelerix albiventris* • African hedgehog • Neoplasia • Cardiomyopathy
- Exotic mammal • Aging • Geriatric

KEY POINTS

- African hedgehogs typically only live 4 to 6 years and are considered geriatric by 3 to 5 years of age. Having such a short life span, they should receive a complete veterinary examination every 6 months.
- Even mild changes in a hedgehog's habits, activity patterns, behavior, weight, eating, or elimination patterns may signal a serious age-related problem. Owners should not ignore these signs or assume that the pet is just slowing down.
- African hedgehogs are particularly susceptible to diseases of the integumentary, gastrointestinal, renal, cardiovascular, and musculoskeletal systems.
- Hedgehogs are prone to neoplasia at an early age. Although it is usually encountered at about 3.5 years of age, neoplasia is reported in hedgehogs as young as 1 month.
- Geriatric hedgehog care should include a low-fat, dry kibble diet; adequate exercise; and regular dental cleaning. Anesthesia in older hedgehogs requires increased vigilance, monitoring, and physiologic support.

INTRODUCTION

Like all exotic pets, the African hedgehog (*Atelerix albiventris*) is susceptible to age-related conditions such as cardiovascular, renal, and periodontal disease. However, hedgehogs are exceptionally short lived and prone to neoplasia, making geriatric hedgehog appointments particularly common in clinical practice. The life expectancy of an African hedgehog is 4 to 6 years, and up to 9 years is recorded.[1,2] If geriatric status is reached at 75% to 80% of usual life span, then African hedgehogs are geriatric by 3 to 5 years of age.[3,4]

EFFECTS OF AGING

The degenerative effects of time gradually lead to progressive, irreversible decreases in organ reserve capacity. At this stage, considered geriatric normal, responses to stress, infection, and drug therapy are altered and serious age-related diseases

Avian and Exotic Animal Care, 8711 Fidelity Boulevard, Raleigh, NC 27617, USA
E-mail address: drdan@avianandexotic.com

Vet Clin Exot Anim 23 (2020) 615–637
https://doi.org/10.1016/j.cvex.2020.05.005
1094-9194/20/© 2020 Elsevier Inc. All rights reserved.

become more prevalent.[3] At some later stage in the gradual decline of an organ, the physiologic tipping point for that organ is eventually reached and its physiologic reserves are exhausted. Signs of borderline organ failure may be subtle, undetected, or misinterpreted by the owner until the patient is stressed by an unrelated illness, boarding, hospitalization, medications, anesthesia, or surgery. This stage is when overt organ failure occurs, and signs become obvious.[5]

SIGNS OF AGING

Hedgehogs are masters at hiding signs of disease. No matter how many generations in captivity, pet hedgehogs are still essentially wild and tend not to attract attention by showing signs of weakness. Owners must closely observe the geriatric hedgehog for early warning signs. Even mild changes in a hedgehog's habits, activity patterns, behavior, weight, eating, or elimination patterns may signal a serious development. They should not write these signs off to old age or assume that nothing can be done (**Box 1**). Owners should report potential problems to the veterinarian as soon as possible. Waiting until the next wellness examination may be too late.[5,6]

Box 1
Signs that may indicate a health problem in the geriatric hedgehog[5,6,32]

Decreased appetite, anorexia

Difficulty eating

Weight loss

Increased water intake

Weakness, ataxia

Lethargy, sleeping excessively

Decreased activity

Diarrhea, abnormal stool

Straining to urinate or defecate

Excessive urination

Vomiting

Drooling

Foul mouth odor

Increased breathing rate or effort

Coughing, sneezing

Loss of fur or spines

Excessive itching

Development of lumps or other skin changes

Obesity/inability to roll up completely

Sudden collapse

Seizure, convulsion (medical emergency)

Evidence of pain

DISEASES OF GERIATRIC HEDGEHOGS

Several retrospective studies of disease occurrence in captive African hedgehogs have recently been undertaken.[2,7,8] These studies indicate that African hedgehogs are especially prone to dermatologic, gastrointestinal, and musculoskeletal diseases.[2] Renal and cardiovascular disease are also common.[9,10] Neoplasia is the most common histologic diagnosis and the most common cause of death in hedgehogs.[7,8] Hedgehogs may be affected by multiple diseases, neoplastic and nonneoplastic, at the same time.[11]

NEOPLASIA

Several reviews of neoplasia in African hedgehogs have been published.[4,12,13] Neoplasia is extremely common and represents the most widely reported disease in hedgehogs.[2,4,14] In retrospective studies of African hedgehogs at necropsy, the prevalence of neoplasia has ranged from 29% to 53%.[9,12,15] When incorporating all body systems, neoplasia was observed in 20.75% (22 of 106) of hedgehogs, making it the third most common general disorder.[2]

A variety of tumors have been identified in hedgehogs, affecting virtually every organ system. The systems most often involved include the integumentary, hemolymphatic, digestive, endocrine, and reproductive systems.[2,4] Epithelial tumors are most prevalent, followed by round cell tumors and mesenchymal or spindle cell tumors.[4] The most common neoplasms encountered in hedgehogs include mammary gland adenocarcinoma, lymphosarcoma, and oral squamous cell carcinoma (SCC).[2,4,13,16] The neoplasia reported most often is oral SCC.[2,7] Finding multiple neoplasms in 1 patient is common.[17–23]

Age is the primary risk factor for neoplasia in African hedgehogs.[4] In a retrospective study of 66 necropsy specimens, the mean age of hedgehogs diagnosed with neoplasia was 3.5 years (range, 2–5.5 years).[12] However, neoplasia is reported in hedgehogs as young as 1 month of age.[15] Risk of neoplasia seems unrelated to gender.[4,13] Although many of the cases referenced here occurred in nongeriatric hedgehogs, they are included in this article because of the association between age and neoplasia in this species.

Clinical signs of neoplasia, if any, depend on the organ systems involved. Neoplasia may be diagnosed incidentally when a patient presents for a different problem. Many cases of neoplasia are diagnosed in chronically debilitated animals presented for urgent care.[14] Evaluation should include a full physical examination under anesthesia, abdominal palpation, thoracic auscultation, and complete oral examination.[4,13] Diagnostic tests to consider include complete blood count (CBC), serum biochemical profile, urinalysis, whole-body radiographs, ultrasonography, fine-needle aspiration cytology, and tissue biopsy. An early and accurate diagnosis is essential for an appropriate prognosis and to provide the best chance for curative treatment.[4,24]

Surgery is the treatment reported and recommended most often for neoplasia in hedgehogs. Complete surgical excision has the potential to be curative in cases of local disease, but it is not effective when there is systemic spread of tumor. Radiotherapy and chemotherapy may also be considered, depending on tumor type and circumstances, but the efficacy of these modalities in the hedgehog is not yet known.[4,16,25] However, neoplasia in African hedgehogs is usually malignant (ie, up to 85% of cases) and tends to carry a poor prognosis.[4,13,16]

RENAL/URINARY

African hedgehogs possess urinary anatomy like that of other small mammals and are susceptible renal disease, urolithiasis, cystitis, and so forth. In an early retrospective review, 14% of lesions (63 of 439) noted at necropsy were found in the urinary system; 49% of these were considered degenerative, 33% inflammatory, and 9% neoplastic.[15] A later study showed histopathologic evidence of renal disease in 50% (7 of 14) of hedgehogs necropsied.[9] A retrospective study of clinical cases identified renal disease in 9.43% of 106 hedgehogs presented to a veterinary teaching hospital.[2] Most cases of degenerative renal disease are reported in patients older than 3 years; however, renal disease has been diagnosed in hedgehogs as young as 7 months.[26]

The histologic diagnoses of kidney disease in African hedgehogs include tubulointerstitial nephritis, chronic renal infarcts, glomerulopathy, tubular nephrosis, glomerulosclerosis, polycystic kidney disease, adenocarcinoma, hemangiosarcoma, and stromal-type nephroblastoma.[9,26,27] Poorly differentiated renal neoplasia is also described.[28] Other reports of urinary tract disease include penile myxoma surgically removed from a hedgehog aged 3 years and 5 months, urethral obstruction caused by accessory gland enlargement in a male hedgehog that was treated by preputial cystostomy, and bilateral renal calculi associated with weight loss, azotemia, and hyperphosphatemia in a geriatric hedgehog.[29–31]

Clinical signs of renal disease in the hedgehog are generally nonspecific and include lethargy, anorexia, dehydration, and weight loss. Observant owners may notice polydipsia and polyuria early in renal disease, with absence of water intake occurring in end-stage renal failure. Depending on where other types of lesions (eg, neoplasia, urolith, infection) occur within the urinary tract hematuria, pyuria, anuria, pollakiuria, and stranguria may be seen.[26,32] Diagnosis of renal and urinary tract disease is confirmed by urinalysis, CBC, and biochemical analysis. Renomegaly, shrunken kidneys, masses, uroliths, and so forth may be seen on radiography and/or ultrasonography.

Long-term subcutaneous fluid therapy is usually indicated in patients with chronic renal failure to diurese and control azotemia and uremia. This process can be particularly difficult in the hedgehog because of its spines and natural defensive behavior of rolling into a tight ball.[26] This problem was overcome in 1 case report where a sterile, fenestrated cannula was placed subcutaneously for long-term fluid administration.[33] Additional treatment of chronic renal failure might include hand feeding, aluminum hydroxide to control hyperphosphatemia, and famotidine or cimetidine to control gastritis.[34] Animals that lose control of urination should be kept on substrate that wicks urine away from the body, thus avoiding scald.[6] The prognosis for geriatric hedgehogs with urinary system disease varies by location and severity, but end-stage renal disease is ultimately fatal.

REPRODUCTIVE

Reproductive disease occurs regularly in geriatric hedgehogs. One retrospective study found reproductive disorders in 8.49% of clinical cases (N = 106).[2] Another found that 5% of hedgehog necropsy lesions (N = 439) affected the reproductive system; 48% of these were considered degenerative, 30% inflammatory, and 22% neoplastic.[15] The types of uterine tumors reported in hedgehogs include adenoleiomyosarcoma, adenosarcoma, endometrial stromal cell sarcoma, endometrial polyps, adenoleiomyoma, uterine adenocarcinoma, carcinosarcoma, and uterine spindle cell tumor.[2,4,13,35–38] Nonneoplastic uterine diseases reported to occur in hedgehogs include uterine hyperplasia, pyometra, and metritis.[2,36] Nonuterine reproductive tumors include vaginal spindle cell tumor, vaginal tunic neurofibrosarcoma, ovarian granulosa cell tumor, malignant ovarian teratoma, and penile myxoma.[4,18,22,29,39–42] There is 1 report of accessory gland enlargement in a male hedgehog that caused urethral obstruction.[30] There is another of hyperplasia of a seminal vesicle identified on histopathology.[8] Risk factors for reproductive disease in African hedgehogs seem to be age and gender.

Clinical signs of reproductive disease in geriatric hedgehogs depend on the organs involved. For uterine disease, vaginal bleeding or other discharge is typical[2,13,14] (**Fig. 1**). For ovarian tumors, clinical signs may include abdominal distension and palpable abdominal mass.[40,41] Hematuria may be the presenting complaint for both uterine disease and granulosa cell tumor. Hematuria may also be a sign of urinary tract disease in either sex.[18,43] Nonspecific signs of reproductive disease can include anorexia and weight loss.[41–43]

Suspicion of reproductive disease is confirmed by the presence of vaginal bleeding or discharge, or by palpation of ovarian mass or enlarged, tubular uterus in the caudoventral abdomen (may require sedation or anesthesia). Diagnosis can involve whole-body radiography, abdominal ultrasonography, CBC, serum biochemical profile, and urinalysis.[4,13] Computed tomography (CT) and cytologic examination of ultrasonography-guided aspirates may be indicated in some cases and exploratory surgery in others.[13,22,35,40]

Treatment of reproductive disease in geriatric hedgehogs is like that in other species. Surgery to remove diseased tissues (uterus, ovary) is curative in most cases[22,42] (**Fig. 2**). In cases of suspected neoplasia, thoracic radiographs are recommended before surgery.[13] Histopathology should be performed on tissues after removal in order to give an accurate prognosis.[13,22] Oral tamoxifen was prescribed postoperatively for 1 hedgehog with granulosa cell tumor and mammary adenocarcinoma, but

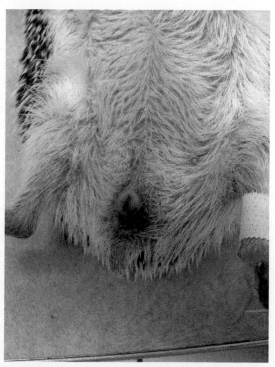

Fig. 1. Vaginal hemorrhage in an African hedgehog. Vaginal bleeding is common with reproductive disease (eg, uterine neoplasia) in geriatric female hedgehogs. Vaginal bleeding may be mistaken for hematuria or hematochezia.

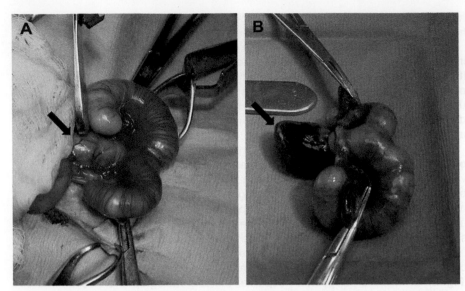

Fig. 2. Uterine tumor in a hedgehog. Uterine disease, particularly neoplasia, is common in geriatric hedgehogs. In the animal pictured, ovariohysterectomy was complicated by a polypoid uterine mass that protruded into the vaginal canal (*arrows*). (*A*) Ventral aspect of diseased uterus before surgical removal. (*B*) Dorsal aspect of same after resection.

attempts to medicate the animal were unsuccessful and drug efficacy could not be assessed.[4]

Prognosis for reproductive disease in geriatric hedgehogs depends on severity at presentation but is usually good. With appropriate therapy, patients are likely to recover. Ovariohysterectomy is the treatment of choice and allows prolonged survival of hedgehogs with uterine neoplasia. Tumors of the uterus are typically histologically low grade and metastasis is rare.[4,43] Many reproductive diseases of the geriatric female hedgehog may be prevented via prophylactic ovariohysterectomy at 6 months of age.

ENDOCRINE

Endocrine disease is rare in geriatric hedgehogs, having a prevalence of less than 2% in 1 report.[2] Of 74 hedgehogs necropsied, endocrine disease comprised 4.6% (20 of 439) of lesions identified in 1 study; 45% of these were classified as neoplastic and 25% as degenerative.[15] Based on previous reports, between 6.7% and 14% of hedgehog tumors are of endocrine origin.[7,44] Even where endocrine neoplasia is diagnosed, clinical signs are rare.[4,13]

Most reports of endocrine disease in African hedgehogs are of endocrine neoplasia. One case of nonneoplastic endocrine disease (thyroid gland hypertrophy) is reported.[2] Endocrine neoplasia reported to date includes thyroid adenocarcinoma, thyroid C-cell carcinoma, thyroid follicular adenoma, thyroid follicular carcinoma, parathyroid adenoma, pancreatic islet cell tumor, pituitary adenoma, pheochromocytoma, adrenal cortical carcinoma, and malignant neuroendocrine tumor.[2,4,12,13,19,45,46]

Endocrine disease in African hedgehogs is often clinically silent.[4,13] Clinical signs, if any, have been nonspecific, including anorexia, weight loss, weakness, and incoordination. A hedgehog later diagnosed with thyroid gland C-cell carcinoma showed dysphagia, weight loss, and tetraparesis.[46] The diagnosis of endocrine disease, which is neoplasia in most cases, is usually made at necropsy and is often incidental.[4,12,13]

Information concerning testing or treatment of endocrine disease in geriatric African hedgehogs is scant. With the current lack of clinical data, it seems reasonable to follow the guidelines used in cats and dogs to formulate appropriate diagnostic and treatment protocols.[4] The prognosis for endocrine disease varies by severity and location. There is 1 report of successful treatment of metastatic C-cell carcinoma with radiation therapy in a geriatric African hedgehog; however, much more work is needed in this area.[45]

NERVOUS

Neurologic disease was identified in 2.7% of necropsy lesions in 1 retrospective study. Of 439 lesions identified, 42% were degenerative, 25% traumatic, 17% vascular, 8% inflammatory, and 8% neoplastic.[15] Causes of neurologic disease include wobbly hedgehog syndrome (WHS), intervertebral disc disease (IVDD), neoplasia, central nervous system (CNS) trauma, toxins, infarcts, malnutrition, otitis media/interna, and torpor.[2] Differential diagnoses to consider include orthopedic trauma, cardiac disease, and arthritis.[16]

WHS is the best-known nervous system disease and the most common cause of ataxia in African hedgehogs.[2] It occurs in approximately 10% of pet African hedgehogs in North America and produces mild ataxia progressing to severe neurologic disease and complete paralysis, usually over a period of several months to a year[47] (**Fig. 3**). Although WHS usually affects animals younger than 2 years of age, it can also occur in older patients.[48,49] On histology, WHS causes vacuolization of the white matter of the brain and spinal cord, with associated neurogenic muscle atrophy without inflammation.[49] Several causes have been proposed, but genetics seem to play a role.[47,50] Treatment is generally unrewarding and has included vitamins E and B, selenium, calcium, prednisone, antibiotics, homeopathic remedies, acupuncture, and physical therapy. No treatment has been shown to halt the progression of paralysis, and euthanasia is eventually indicated.[14,47] WHS may occur in conjunction with cardiac and other diseases.[48]

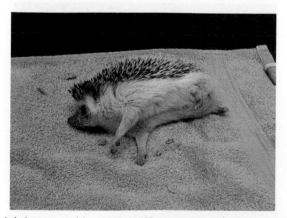

Fig. 3. Difficulty righting caused by WHS. WHS causes neurologic symptoms ranging from mild ataxia to complete paralysis over several months to a year or more. Most affected hedgehogs are less than 2 years of age, but geriatric hedgehogs are also sometimes affected. WHS occurs in about 10% of African hedgehogs in North America.

IVDD is common in geriatric hedgehogs and can present with clinical signs resembling WHS, including progressive hind-limb ataxia, urinary stasis, loss of proprioception, and lameness.[2,51] Radiographic findings associated with IVDD include spondylosis deformans, intervertebral disc space narrowing, and intervertebral disc mineralization.[51,52] Spondylosis deformans is a common incidental finding on hedgehog radiographs and not always associated with clinical disease (see **Fig. 5**). IVDD has been reported in conjunction with fatal herpes simplex type 1 infection.[53]

Neoplasia of the CNS may cause clinical signs such as WHS and IVDD.[54–58] CNS tumors reported in hedgehogs include soft tissue sarcoma, histiocytic sarcoma, ganglioglioma, gemistocytic astrocytoma, oligodendroglioma, anaplastic astrocytoma, microglioma, oligoastrocytoma, meningioma, and lymphoma.[2,54,56–61]

Clinical signs of neurologic disease most often include ataxia, loss of balance, and paresis/paralysis.[2,32] Circling can be caused by otitis media/interna or primary neurologic disease.[2] Seizures (in association with a brain tumor) have also been reported.[57] Diagnosis is usually made through radiography, ultrasonography, CT, MRI, or necropsy.[51,52,61,62] Treatment of neurologic disease is often unrewarding. Prognosis for WHS and neoplasia is ultimately poor, whereas hedgehogs with IVDD may experience temporary relief with nonsteroidal antiinflammatory drugs (NSAIDs) and analgesics. The prognosis for hedgehogs with bacterial otitis interna/media is usually good with appropriate treatment (NSAIDs, antibiotics).

OPHTHALMIC

Reports of ophthalmic disease in geriatric African hedgehogs include neoplasia, exophthalmos, proptosis, and injury. Intraocular hemangioma is reported, as is exophthalmos secondary to neoplasia.[4,57,63,64] Hedgehogs may be predisposed to proptosis because of shallow orbits (**Fig. 4**). Eight cases of unilateral proptosis revealed histopathologic lesions including orbital cellulitis, panophthalmitis, and corneal ulceration.[65] Ocular injuries may be difficult to treat even with aggressive medical management, because most hedgehogs do not tolerate repeated topical application of ocular medication. Enucleation may be required and is well tolerated because vision is less

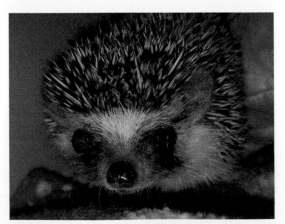

Fig. 4. Bilateral proptosis in an African hedgehog. Hedgehogs may be predisposed to exophthalmos, proptosis, and ocular injury because of their prominent eyes and shallow orbits. Disease may be unilateral or bilateral. Causes include neoplasia, infection, trauma, and inflammation; however, many times the cause is unknown.

important to hedgehogs than hearing or smell.[16,66] Cataracts were reported in 3.77% (N = 106) of clinical cases in 1 report.[2] There are no reports of glaucoma, retinopathy, or other ophthalmic conditions in African hedgehogs.

HEMOLYMPHATIC

Hematopoietic disease represented 18.5% of necropsy lesions in 1 retrospective study.[15] Hemolymphatic neoplasia accounts for approximately 11% of hedgehog tumors, making this system the second most likely to be affected by neoplasia.[12] Lymphoma is the second most common tumor of the hedgehog overall and occurs in both multicentric and gastrointestinal forms.[4,13,61] A retroviral origin for some cases has been suggested.[67] Other forms of hemolymphatic neoplasia in African hedgehogs include myelogenous leukemia, eosinophilic leukemia, intestinal plasmacytoma, multiple myeloma, histiocytic sarcoma, and malignant neuroendocrine tumor (carcinoid) of the spleen.[4,22,23,30,56,68–72] Splenic extramedullary hematopoiesis seems to be common.[9,37]

Clinical signs of hemolymphatic neoplasia are often nonspecific but may reflect the organ systems affected. CBC is frequently important in the diagnosis. Serum biochemistry may be unremarkable, but changes may reflect organ involvement.[4] Diagnosis of hemolymphatic disease is possible by radiography, ultrasonography, CT, MRI, exploratory surgery, fine-needle aspirate, soft tissue biopsy, bone marrow biopsy, cytology, and histopathology. A definitive antemortem diagnosis of hemolymphatic cancer is atypical because most cases are diagnosed at necropsy.[30] The efficacy of chemotherapy is unknown, and surgery may be curative in rare cases.[4,30] Prognosis is generally poor.

CARDIOVASCULAR

Cardiovascular disease is common in African hedgehogs. However, retrospective studies differ on the prevalence. One study found cardiac disease in 1.89% of 106 clinical cases, whereas another found that 8% (35 of 439) of necropsy lesions were cardiovascular, and a third found cardiomyopathy in 38% of 42 postmortem cases.[2,10,15] Most cardiovascular lesions (68%) are degenerative.[15] Geriatric males are more likely to have cardiac disease but reports of affected animals include those as young as 1 year of age.[73] Reports of cardiovascular disease in the literature include cardiomyopathy, valvular endocardiosis, and bilateral atrial thrombosis.[10,11,48,74] Vascular thrombosis, including saddle thrombus, is also reported.[37] Reports of cardiovascular neoplasia are rare.[4]

Possible causes of cardiac disease in the African hedgehog include diet, toxin, stress, obesity, and genetics.[73] Carnitine deficiency may promote cardiomyopathy in geriatric hedgehogs.[74] Clinical signs of cardiovascular disease in hedgehogs include heart murmur, lethargy, general weakness, icterus, moist rales, anorexia, cyanosis, tachypnea, dyspnea, exercise intolerance, dehydration, collapse, and weight loss. Acute death without clinical signs is also reported.[10,32,48,74,75] Heart murmurs can be difficult to detect in a moving hedgehog, especially one that is snuffling or grunting, as is common on examination. Heart disease may therefore not be detected until it is in the advanced stages.[75]

Diagnosis of cardiovascular disease is possible via radiography, ultrasonography, electrocardiogram (ECG), and necropsy.[14,76] Normal cardiac parameters for radiographic cardiac measurement, echocardiogram, and ECG in African hedgehogs have been established.[75] Radiographic findings associated with cardiac disease include enlarged heart, pulmonary edema, aerophagia, tracheal elevation, pleural edema, and pleural effusion.[73,74] On ultrasonography, a fractional shortening of less than 25% has been reported as consistent with cardiac dysfunction.[1] Necropsy findings include cardiomegaly, hepatomegaly, pulmonary edema or congestion, hydrothorax, ascites, and pulmonary or renal infarcts.[73] Histopathologic lesions in 1 study were mainly associated with the left ventricular myocardium and included myodegeneration, myonecrosis, atrophy, hypertrophy, and myofiber disarray.[10] Myocardial mineralization or calcinosis has been described as a necropsy finding in pet hedgehogs with concurrent diseases, the clinical significance of which is not known.[37,64]

Treatments to consider for cardiovascular disease in African hedgehogs include furosemide, enalapril, pimobendan, digoxin, and L-carnitine.[14,34,48,74,76] The overall prognosis is reported to be poor; however, successful emergency treatment of congestive heart failure has been reported.[14,74]

RESPIRATORY

Primary respiratory disease is common in African hedgehogs, representing 8.9% of necropsy lesions in 1 retrospective study. In that study, 49% of respiratory lesions were degenerative and 41% were inflammatory.[15] Pneumonia was identified in 14% of hedgehogs necropsied in another report.[9] In a third investigation, respiratory disease was at least partly responsible for 25.6% of hedgehog deaths.[7] Hedgehogs are susceptible to respiratory infection by *Bordetella bronchiseptica*, *Pasteurella multocida*, and *Corynebacterium* species.[77] There is 1 report of an African hedgehog with disseminated histoplasmosis.[78] Fatal bronchopneumonia caused by skunk adenovirus 1 is also reported.[79] Pneumonia is generally more common in hedgehogs that are old, debilitated, and have concurrent disease. Reports of neoplasia in the respiratory system include SCC of the oral and nasal cavities, bronchoalveolar carcinoma of the lung, osteosarcoma of a rib, and various metastatic pulmonary tumors.[4,12,13,64,80]

Clinical signs of respiratory disease include dyspnea, stertor, sneezing, wheezing, nasal discharge, exercise intolerance, and abdominal breathing.[16,32] It can be difficult to differentiate the normal snuffling noises that a hedgehog may make from true dyspnea.[16] Dyspnea associated with pulmonary neoplasia can mimic pneumonia or heart disease.[77]

Diagnosis of respiratory disease includes nasal cytology, culture, and sensitivity; head and thoracic radiology, CT, or MRI; and tracheal wash cytology, culture, and sensitivity[16,77] (**Fig. 5**). CBC may reflect changes consistent with infection in cases of bacterial pneumonia. Nonrespiratory causes of dyspnea, such as cardiac disease, should also be ruled out.[16] Treatment of bacterial infection is systemic antibiotics and nebulization based on culture and sensitivity. The hedgehog's shy nature and tendency to roll when threatened make oral medications less attractive than injections and nebulization therapy.[77] Prognosis for respiratory disease in geriatric hedgehogs depends on location and cause. Although treatment of neoplasia is usually unrewarding, bacterial respiratory infections are often treatable.

DIGESTIVE

In a retrospective review of 74 African hedgehog necropsies, more lesions (32%) were found in the digestive system than any other system. Forty-four percent of these were considered inflammatory, 39% degenerative, and 7% neoplastic.[15] The gastrointestinal tract is the third most common site of neoplastic disease in the hedgehog, accounting for 16% of reported tumors.[12,44]

Oral SCC is the most common tumor of the African hedgehog digestive system and is also the most common overall neoplasia according to recent reports[2,7] (**Fig. 6**). Affected animals may be male or female and aged from 1 to 6 years.[2,12] Other

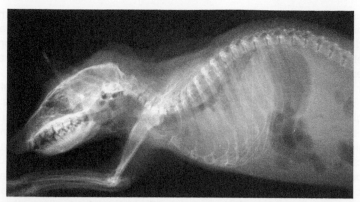

Fig. 5. Pneumonia and spondylosis deformans in an African hedgehog. Radiographic signs of pneumonia in this patient include alveolar pattern and air bronchogram, and differential diagnosis would include heart failure. Multifocal curvilinear mineralizations are visible ventral to the last few thoracic and first lumbar intervertebral disk spaces. Although these may represent spondylosis (sometimes associated with IVDD), they are a common incidental finding in normal hedgehogs. They are so common that some radiologists do not consider them to be spondylosis lesions; these hemal arches may be a common variant in African hedgehogs (Maria Evola, DVM, DACVR, personal communication, 2020).

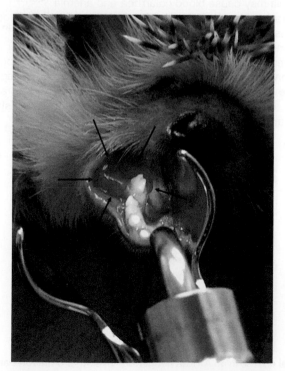

Fig. 6. Oral tumor in an African hedgehog. Oral tumors like this (*black arrows*) are particularly common in geriatric African hedgehogs. Squamous cell carcinoma and other oral neoplasms occur frequently. The primary differential for these is periodontal disease, which is also common.

digestive system neoplasms include oral fibrosarcoma, odontogenic fibroma, osteoma, acinic cell carcinoma, pleomorphic salivary adenoma, intestinal plasmacytoma, gastric adenocarcinoma, intestinal adenocarcinoma, intestinal lymphosarcoma, metastatic colonic mucinous adenocarcinoma, pancreatic exocrine carcinoma, and metastatic hepatocellular carcinoma.[4,12,25,63,64,67,69,81–83]

African hedgehogs are particularly susceptible to gingivitis, dental calculus, periodontitis, and loss of teeth (**Fig. 7**). The prevalence of these in 1 study was 4.72%.[2] Free-ranging hedgehogs are similarly affected.[84] Hedgehogs with dental disease often develop profound gingival hyperplasia that is similar in appearance to neoplasia and should be distinguished from it with histopathology.[62,81] Nuts, grains, and other hard items (eg, peanuts) should be avoided, because they may wedge against the palate and become a foreign body.[1,32] Hedgehogs are also susceptible to oral trauma and osteomyelitis.[62] Other nonneoplastic digestive system diseases include enteritis (including *Salmonella* spp infection), gastrointestinal foreign body obstruction, and hepatic lipidosis.[7,14,16,67]

Clinical signs of digestive disease depend on lesion location and severity. For dental disease and/or oral neoplasia, these include reduced food intake, change in food preference, anorexia, weight loss, dysphagia, drooling, presence of blood, and/or foul breath.[62,81] There may be gingival swelling and inflammation, loose teeth, tooth loss, orofacial swellings, or deviation of jaw bones.[44,80,81] Signs of gastrointestinal disease in the hedgehog include inappetence, weight loss, diarrhea, malodorous feces, decreased quantity or frequency of defecation, and vomiting.[32,62] In addition, gastrointestinal neoplasia may cause bloody diarrhea and anemia.[14,67,83]

Diagnosis of oral and dental disease is based on tissue biopsy/histopathology, bacterial culture/sensitivity, radiography, CT, and other imaging.[4,52,81,85] Fine-needle aspiration and impression smear cytology may be diagnostic, but alone are often insufficient.[4,86] Periodontal disease in its early stages can resemble oral SCC cytologically, thus caution must be taken when evaluating such lesions.[24] Diagnosis of gastrointestinal disease is based on fecal examination, CBC/chemistry, radiography, and ultrasonography. Exploratory laparotomy, surgical biopsy, and histopathology are sometimes indicated.[87]

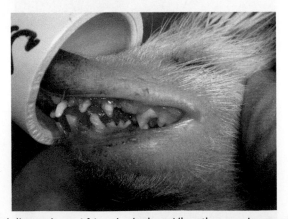

Fig. 7. Periodontal disease in an African hedgehog. Like other omnivores and carnivores, African hedgehogs are susceptible to periodontal disease, including gingivitis, dental calculus, periodontitis, and loss of teeth. Periodontal disease may be preventable with proper diet. A diet of dry kibble and uncooked fruits and vegetables may help prevent periodontal disease, whereas moist or canned foods tend to promote it.

Surgical removal of hedgehog oral tumors can be attempted, but removal of the entire tumor may be difficult, and a high rate of reoccurrence is reported. If treatment is attempted, follow-up with chemotherapy, radiation, or cryotherapy under the guidance of a veterinary oncologist should be considered.[4,62,86] Electrochemotherapy for oral SCC using intralesional bleomycin injection followed by trains of biphasic electric pulses provided partial remission for 5 months in 1 report.[88] Another report describes successful surgical removal of peripheral odontogenic fibromas without relapse.[25] The placement, maintenance, and successful use of an esophagostomy tube to manage severe oral trauma in a hedgehog has been described.[89]

Gingivitis and periodontitis are likely to respond to appropriate antibiotic therapy. Loose and infected teeth should be removed, and osteomyelitis should be aggressively treated. Bacterial culture/sensitivity and histopathology are likely to provide important information.[16,81,85] Gastrointestinal illnesses can be treated with the same supportive care, dietary manipulations, antibiotics, antiparasitics, antacids, and gastroprotectants as for ferrets, dogs, and cats.[34,87]

The prognosis for most cases of hedgehog oral and gastrointestinal neoplasia is poor. The prognosis for periodontal and other nonneoplastic diseases of the digestive system is fair to good. Dental disease in geriatric hedgehogs may be preventable by offering hard kibble or uncooked produce rather than moist or canned food.[16,32,90]

INTEGUMENTARY

Diseases of the integument are the most prevalent health disorders of African hedgehogs, affecting 66% of patients. *Caparinia* or *Chorioptes* spp mite infestations are the most reported skin problem, but *Notoedres cati* is also occasionally diagnosed.[1,2] Dermatophytosis with either *Trichophyton* or *Microsporum* spp is also common, and concurrent mite/dermatophyte infections are common. Dermatophytes may be carried asymptomatically and are a zoonotic risk.[2,16] Viral papillomatosis and bacterial dermatitis are also reported.[91,92] Bite wounds and other injuries to the skin, sometimes with secondary infection or abscessation, pododermatitis, and otitis externa, are possible.[2] Pinnal dermatitis, which causes the margins of the pinna to appear ragged or crusty, is a benign condition often seen in older hedgehogs (**Fig. 8**). Possible causes include dermatophytes, acariasis, nutritional deficiencies, dry skin, seborrhea with hyperkeratosis, accumulated skin secretions, and extension of ear canal disease.[1]

The integument is frequently affected by neoplasia in geriatric hedgehogs.[2,12] Reported histologic types include nerve sheath tumors (schwannoma or neurofibrosarcoma), neurofibroma, malignant fibrous histiocytoma, plasmacytoma, lymphoma, hemangiosarcoma, fibrosarcoma, osteosarcoma, undifferentiated or poorly differentiated sarcomas, sebaceous carcinoma, lipoma, liposarcoma, SCC, mast cell tumors, and mammary gland tumors.[4,17,18,21,38,93–101] Mammary gland adenocarcinoma was the single most common neoplasm affecting African hedgehogs in 1 report.[4] Mammary tumors are most likely to occur in female hedgehogs greater than 3 years of age, are usually malignant, and may metastasize.[4,62]

Clinical signs of integumentary disease include excessive flaking or crusting of skin or spines; dirty, crusty, or itchy ears; head shaking; itching; scratching; losing spines; and lumps or bumps on or just under the skin, or involving the mammary glands.[32] Diagnosis usually involves skin scrape, bacterial and/or fungal culture, impression smear cytology, fine-needle aspirate and/or cytology, and skin biopsy.[24,92,95]

Treatment of skin infection is with appropriate antimicrobial or antiparasitic medications. Prognosis for recovery is usually good. Treatment of integumentary neoplasia is

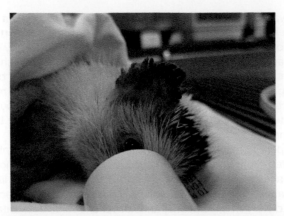

Fig. 8. Pinnal dermatitis in a geriatric hedgehog. Pinnal dermatitis is a benign condition of older hedgehogs that causes the margins of the pinna to become ragged or crusty. Possible causes include dermatophytosis, acariasis, nutritional deficiencies, dry skin, seborrhea with hyperkeratosis, accumulated skin secretions, and extension of otitis externa.

with surgery if complete resection is possible; however, metastatic skin tumors are common, and most mammary tumors are malignant. Prognosis varies by tumor type.[4]

MUSCULOSKELETAL

Musculoskeletal disease in the hedgehog comprised 4.6% of necropsy lesions in 1 survey. Of these lesions, 55% were inflammatory, 20% degenerative, and 20% traumatic.[15] The prevalence of musculoskeletal disease among hedgehog clinical cases was more than 15% in another report and included conditions such as obesity (10.38%), degenerative joint disease (1.89%), spondylosis (2.83%), and annular pedal constriction (4.72%)[2] (**Figs. 9** and **10**). Most reports of musculoskeletal neoplasia in hedgehogs concern osteosarcoma.[4,20,102–104] Multicentric skeletal sarcomas (associated with probable retrovirus particles) and anaplastic fibrosarcoma have also been reported.[64,105] Other musculoskeletal problems include trauma from falls and other injuries, which occur frequently in hedgehogs because of their tendency to climb and explore their environment.[14,16,106]

Clinical signs of musculoskeletal disease include lameness, inactivity, swelling, bruising, and other evidence of trauma.[32] Diagnosis typically involves radiography or CT imaging.[52,104,107] CBC and chemistry may aid in some diagnoses. In cases of neoplasia, impression smears, fine-needle aspirate cytology, and histopathology may also be indicated.[4,24,93,102] Orthopedic treatments for fracture or dislocation may be attempted, although stabilization of a limb can be challenging in patients whose automatic response is to roll up. Treatment often involves surgery, and, if amputation of a limb is indicated, hedgehogs seem to cope well.[16,93,108,109] Prognosis depends on severity and location; however, musculoskeletal disease as a cause of death is rare.[7]

GERIATRIC HEDGEHOG CARE

Senior hedgehogs need a balanced, high-protein, low-fat, commercial dry kibble (hedgehog, insectivore, low-fat cat or dog food) to prevent obesity and maintain dental health. Limit the volume of food offered, feed only at night, and remove any uneaten

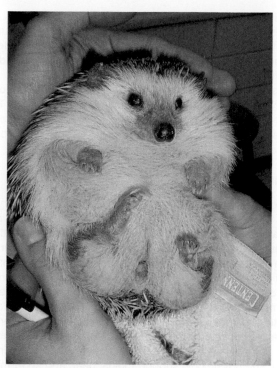

Fig. 9. Obese African hedgehog. Obesity in captive hedgehogs is common. It can be so severe as to prevent a hedgehog from rolling into defensive posture and may contribute to heart disease. Obesity may be prevented by offering a low-fat diet, limiting the quantity of food provided, and encouraging exercise and normal foraging behavior.

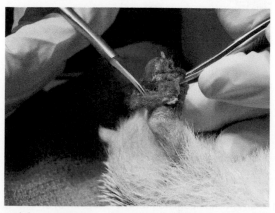

Fig. 10. Annular pedal constriction. Constricting injury is frequently encountered in African hedgehogs, and multiple limbs may be affected. Annular constriction may occur when a limb becomes entrapped in hair or fibers, resulting in local congestion, edema, hypoxia, and/or avascular necrosis. Frayed towels and human hairs are often responsible.

food in the morning. Although uncooked fruits and vegetables may help to prevent periodontal disease, moist or canned foods should be avoided because they promote it. Insect-only diets should be avoided because these are calcium deficient and promote nutritional secondary hyperparathyroidism. Fresh water should be freely available in either a drinking bottle or shallow bowl.[16,32,90]

Daily exercise should be encouraged (ie, running wheel, time out of cage, foraging box, hunting for live insects). Supplemental heat (eg, heat lamp over 1 corner of cage) that provides a microclimate between 25°C and 30°C (75°F–85°F) is recommended. Temperatures less than 15.6°C (60°F) may induce torpor, which decreases metabolism and resistance to infection, and should be avoided.[2,32]

ANESTHETIC CONSIDERATIONS

Anesthetic risk increases with age. Decreased cardiac and respiratory function, blood pressure control, thermoregulatory ability, and renal and other organ reserve capacity make geriatric patients less able to cope with the stresses of anesthesia. Even mild anesthetic depression, which is not a problem for younger patients, can lead to adverse events in older individuals.[3] Despite these risks, anesthesia is frequently indicated because of the tendency of hedgehogs to roll up when threatened. Inhalant gas (isoflurane or sevoflurane) is the preferred anesthetic for physical examinations, venipuncture, radiography, and other routine procedures. A large canine face mask can be used as an induction chamber in most cases. Endotracheal intubation provides better airway control than a mask and is recommended for surgery and procedures lasting longer than 15 to 20 minutes[110] (**Fig. 11**). Geriatric hedgehogs require increased vigilance, monitoring, and physiologic support (fluids, heat, and so forth) compared with younger animals.[3,32]

GERIATRIC PREVENTIVE CARE

The life span of hedgehogs is short, so the author recommends wellness physical examinations on a 6-month basis. Weight (in grams) should be recorded at every visit.

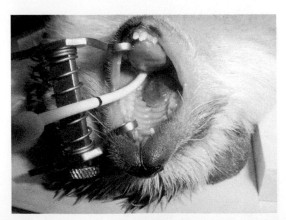

Fig. 11. Intubation of an African hedgehog for the resection of an oral tumor. Endotracheal intubation provides better control of the patient's airway than a mask and is recommended for anesthetic procedures lasting longer than 15 to 20 minutes. Intubation facilitates surgery of the head and oral cavity, dentistry, anesthetic monitoring, and tracheal wash in exotic companion mammals. The author uses a 1.0-mm semiflexible fiberscope and 1.5-mm straight silicone endotracheal tube to intubate hedgehogs.

Full clinical examination (especially to assess the oral cavity and abdomen) generally requires sedation or general anesthesia. To detect gradual physiologic deteriorations in organ function before they become serious, geriatric hedgehogs should also receive wellness CBC, chemistry profile, fecal examination, and urinalysis at least annually. Where indicated, more frequent physical examination or additional diagnostics (ultrasonography, radiographs, and so forth) may be recommended.[4–6]

MANAGING CHRONIC PAIN

Like other senior pets, geriatric hedgehogs are susceptible to chronic pain from injuries, arthritis, dental disease, and so on. African hedgehogs are treated with many of the same analgesics and nutraceuticals as canines and felines. Most dosages are based on anecdotal evidence or extrapolated from other carnivores. Persuading a hedgehog to take oral medications can be difficult. Some of the veterinary compounding kits may be useful in providing flavoring that a hedgehog may like, such as fruit flavors.[32]

EUTHANASIA

Indications for euthanasia in geriatric African hedgehogs include lack of appetite, inability to move well, signs of pain and/or other quality-of-life issues, lack of response to owner interaction, poor prognosis, and owner finances. To minimize patient stress, catheter placement before euthanasia is not usually recommended. Euthanasia usually consists of premedication with either inhalant gas or an overdose of an intramuscular sedative injection followed by injection of sodium pentobarbital or a similar agent.[6,62]

SUMMARY

African hedgehogs have a short life span and are thus considered geriatric by 3 to 5 years. They are susceptible to many of the same geriatric conditions as other carnivores and omnivores, but they are especially prone to neoplasia. Because they are often shy and secretive, it is particularly important for veterinarians to perform a complete physical examination on geriatric hedgehogs every 6 to 12 months using anesthesia or sedation if indicated. By diagnosing age-related conditions as early as possible, better medical and surgical outcomes may be achieved, and a better quality of life may be provided for the geriatric hedgehog patient.

DISCLOSURE

The author has nothing to disclose.

REFERENCES

1. Ivey E, Carpenter JW. African hedgehogs. In: Quesenberry K, Carpenter J, editors. Ferrets, rabbits, and rodents: clinical medicine and surgery. 3rd edition. St Louis (MO): Elsevier Saunders; 2012. p. 411–27.
2. Gardhouse S, Eshar D. Retrospective study of disease occurrence in captive African pygmy hedgehogs (*Atelerix albiventris*). Isr J Vet Med 2015;70(1):32–6.
3. Harvey RC, Paddleford RR. Management of geriatric patients: a common occurrence. Vet Clin North Am Small Anim Pract 1999;29(3):683–99.
4. Heatley JJ, Mauldin GE, Cho DY. A review of neoplasia in the captive African hedgehog (*Atelerix albiventris*). Semin Avian Exot Pet Med 2005;14(3):182–92.

5. Fortney WD. Implementing a successful senior/geriatric health care program for veterinarians, veterinary technicians, and office managers. Vet Clin North Am Small Anim Pract 2012;42(4):823–34.

6. Fisher PG. Exotic mammal geriatrics. Proc Western Veterinary Conference 2011. Available at: https://www.vin.com/members/cms/project/defaultadv1.aspx?id=5183519&pid=11324&. Accessed November 12, 2019.

7. Pei-Chi H, Jane-Fang Y, Lih-Chiann W. A retrospective study of the medical status on 63 African hedgehogs (*Atelerix Albiventris*) at the Taipei zoo from 2003 to 2011. J Exot Pet Med 2015;24:105–11.

8. Okada K, Kondo H, Sumi A, et al. A retrospective study of disease incidence in African pygmy hedgehogs (*Atelerix albiventris*). J Vet Med Sci 2018;80(10):1504–10.

9. Raymond JT, White MR. Necropsy and histopathologic findings in 14 African hedgehogs (*Atelerix albiventris*): a retrospective study. J Zoo Wildl Med 1999;30(2):273–7.

10. Raymond JT, Garner MM. Cardiomyopathy in captive African hedgehogs (*Atelerix albiventris*). J Vet Diagn Invest 2000;12(5):468–72.

11. Yarto E, Fajardo J, Morales M, et al. Bilateral atrial thrombosis in an African hedgehog (Atelerix albiventris) with cardiomyopathy, endometrial hyperplasia and left cystic ovary. J Exot Pet Med, in press.

12. Raymond JT, Garner MM. Spontaneous tumours in captive African hedgehogs (*Atelerix albiventris*): a retrospective study. J Comp Pathol 2001;124:128–33.

13. Greenacre CB. Spontaneous tumors of small mammals. Vet Clin North Am Exot Anim Pract 2004;7(3):627–51.

14. Lennox A. Emergency and critical care procedures in sugar gliders (*Petaurus breviceps*), African hedgehogs (*Atelerix albiventris*) and prairie dogs (*Cynomys spp*). Vet Clin North Am Exot Anim Pract 2007;10(2):533–55.

15. Done LB, Dietze M, Cranfield M, et al. Necropsy lesions by body systems in African hedgehogs (Atelerix albiventris): clues to clinical diagnosis. Proc of Annual Meeting of American Association of Zoo Veterinarians. Oakland, CA, November 15-19, 1992. p. 110–12.

16. Hedley J. African pygmy hedgehogs: general care and health concerns. Companion Animal 2014;19(1):40–4.

17. Raymond J, Garner M. Mammary gland tumors in captive African hedgehogs. J Wildl Dis 2000;36:405–8.

18. Wellehan JF, Southorn E, Smith DA, et al. Surgical removal of a mammary adenocarcinoma and a granulosa cell tumor in an African pygmy hedgehog. Can Vet J 2003;44(3):235–7.

19. Juan-Sallés C, Raymond JT, Garner MM, et al. Adrenocortical carcinoma in three captive African hedgehogs (*Atelerix albiventris*). J Exot Pet Med 2006;15(4):278–80.

20. Rhody JL, Schiller CA. Spinal osteosarcoma in a hedgehog with pedal self-mutilation. Vet Clin North Am Exot Anim Pract 2006;9(3):625–31.

21. Matute AR, Bernal AM, Lezama JR, et al. Sebaceous gland carcinoma and mammary gland carcinoma in an African hedgehog (*Atelerix albiventris*). J Zoo Wildl Med 2014;45(3):682–5.

22. Higbie C, Eshar D, Choudhary S, et al. Eosinophilic leukemia in a pet African hedgehog (*Atelerix albiventris*). J Exot Pet Med 2016;25(1):65–71.

23. Escobar-Alarcón DJ, Reyes-Matute A, Méndez-Bernal A, et al. Chronic eosinophilic leukemia in an African hedgehog (*Atelerix albiventris*). Braz J Vet Pathol 2016;9(1):34–8.

24. Juan-Sallés C, Garner MM. Cytologic diagnosis of diseases of hedgehogs. Vet Clin North Am Exot Anim Pract 2007;10(1):51–9.

25. Wozniak-Biel A, Janeczek M, Janus I, et al. Surgical resection of peripheral odontogenic fibromas in African pygmy hedgehog (Atelerix albiventris): a case study. BMC Vet Res 2015;11:145.

26. Fisher PG. Exotic mammal renal disease: causes and clinical presentation. Vet Clin North Am Exot Anim Pract 2006;9(1):33–67.

27. Ueda K, Imada T, Ueda A, et al. Stromal-type nephroblastoma with or without anaplasia in two hedgehogs (Atelerix albiventris). J Comp Pathol 2019;172: 48–52.

28. Harrison TM, Kitchell BE. Principles and applications of medical oncology in exotic animals. Vet Clin North Am Exot Anim Pract 2017;20(1):209–34.

29. Takami Y, Yasuda N, Une Y. Myxoma of the penis in an African pygmy hedgehog (Atelerix albiventris). J Vet Med Sci 2017;79(1):171–4.

30. Koizumi I, Kondo H. Clinical management and outcome of four-toed hedgehogs (Atelerix albiventris) with histiocytic sarcoma. J Vet Med Sci 2019;81(4):545–50.

31. Johnson DH. Hedgehog with suspected bilateral renal calculi. Exotic DVM 2001; 3(1):5.

32. Simone-Freilicher EA, Hoefer HL. Hedgehog care and husbandry. Vet Clin North Am Exot Anim Pract 2004;7(2):257–67.

33. Powers LV. Subcutaneous implantable catheter for fluid administration in an African pygmy hedgehog. Exot DVM 2002;4(5):16–7.

34. Helmer PJ, Carpenter J. Hedgehogs. In: Carpenter J, Marion C, editors. Exotic animal formulary. 4th edition. St Louis (MO): Saunders; 2012. p. 443–58.

35. Done B, Deem SL, Fiorello CV. Surgical and medical management of a uterine spindle cell tumor in an African hedgehog (Atelerix albiventris). J Zoo Wildl Med 2007;38(4):601–3.

36. Chambers JK, Shiga T, Takimoto H, et al. Proliferative lesions of the endometrium of 50 four-toed hedgehogs (Atelerix albiventris). Vet Pathol 2018;55(4): 562–71.

37. Allison N. A hyperplastic endometrial polyp and vascular thrombosis in a hedgehog. Vet Med 2003;98(4):298–303.

38. Tsai FY, Chang HM, Chang HK, et al. Case report: endometrial stromal sarcoma and liposarcoma in an African hedgehog (Atelerix albiventris). Taiwan Vet J 2019;42(3):181–6.

39. Ramos-Vara JA. Soft tissue sarcomas in the African hedgehog (Atelerix albiventris): microscopic and immunohistologic study of three cases. J Vet Diagn Invest 2001;13(5):442–5.

40. Song SH, Park NW, Jung SK, et al. Bilateral malignant ovarian teratoma with peritoneal metastasis in a captive African pygmy hedgehog (Atelerix albiventris). J Exot Pet Med 2014;23(4):403–8.

41. Bitzmann-Schleiderl D, Ludwig E. Granulosa cell tumor in an African pygmy hedgehog (Atelerix albiventris). Kleintierpraxis 2017;62(9):536–44.

42. Lazarz B, Rother N. Bilateral granulosa cell tumor and hyperplastic uterine pathology in an African pygmy hedgehog (Atelerix albiventris). Kleintierpraxis 2019;64(2):56–63.

43. Mikaelian I, Reavill DR. Spontaneous proliferative lesions and tumors of the uterus of captive African hedgehogs (Atelerix albiventris). J Zoo Wildl Med 2004;35(2):216–20.

44. Raymond JT, Garner MM: Spontaneous tumors in hedgehogs: a retrospective study of fifty cases. Proc Joint Conf American Association of Zoo Veterinarians,

American Association of Wildlife Veterinarians, Association of Reptilian and Amphibian Veterinarians, and National Association of Zoo and Wildlife Veterinarians. Oakland, CA, September 18-23, 2001. p. 326-7.

45. LaRue MK, Flesner BK, Higbie CT, et al. Treatment Of a thyroid tumor in an African Pygmy hedgehog (*Atelerix albiventris*). J Exot Pet Med 2016;25:226-30.

46. Miller DL, Styer EL, Stobaeus JK, et al. Thyroid C-cell carcinoma in an African pygmy hedgehog (*Atelerix albiventris*). J Zoo Wildl Med 2002;33(4):392-6.

47. Graesser D, Spraker TR, Dressen P, et al. Wobbly hedgehog syndrome in African pygmy hedgehogs (*Atelerix spp.*). J Exot Pet Med 2006;15(1):59-65.

48. Hedley J, Benato L, Fraga G, et al. Congestive heart failure due to endocardiosis of the mitral valves in an African pygmy hedgehog. J Exot Pet Med 2013; 22(2):212-7.

49. Díaz-Delgado J, Whitley DB, Storts RW, et al. The pathology of wobbly hedgehog syndrome. Vet Pathol 2018;55(5):711-8.

50. Oliveira LB, Lóes Moreira MV, de Magalhães Santos WH, et al. Wobbly syndrome in an African pygmy hedgehog (*Atelerix albiventris*): neuropathological and immunohistochemical studies. Cienc Rural 2019;49(1):1-6.

51. Raymond JT, Aguilar R, Dunker F, et al. Intervertebral disc disease in African hedgehogs (*Atelerix albiventris*): four cases. J Exot Pet Med 2009;18(3):220-3.

52. Grosso FV. Orthopedic diagnostic imaging in exotic pets. Vet Clin North Am Exot Anim Pract 2019;22(2):149-73.

53. Allison N, Chang T, Steele K, et al. Fatal herpes simplex infection in a pygmy African hedgehog (*Atelerix albiventris*). J Comp Pathol 2002;126(1):76-81.

54. Díaz-Delgado J, Pool R, Hoppes S, et al. Spontaneous multicentric soft tissue sarcoma in a captive African pygmy hedgehog (*Atelerix albiventris*): case report and literature review. J Vet Med Sci 2017;79(5):889-95.

55. Nakata M, Miwa Y, Itou T, et al. Astrocytoma in an African hedgehog (*Atelerix albiventris*) suspected wobbly hedgehog syndrome. J Vet Med Sci 2011; 73(10):1333-5.

56. Ogihara K, Suzuki K, Madarame H. Primary histiocytic sarcoma of the brain in an African hedgehog (*Atelerix albiventris*). J Comp Pathol 2017;157(4):241-5.

57. Kondo H, Yamamoto N, Seino N, et al. Cerebral meningioma in an African pygmy hedgehog (*Atelerix Albiventris*). J Exot Pet Med 2019;28(1):56-8.

58. Gibson CJ, Parry NM, Jakowski RM, et al. Anaplastic astrocytoma in the spinal cord of an African pygmy hedgehog (*Atelerix albiventris*). Vet Pathol 2008;45(6): 934-8.

59. Muñoz-Gutiérrez JF, Garner MM, Kiupel M. Primary central nervous system neoplasms in African hedgehogs. J Vet Diagn Invest 2018;30(5):715-20.

60. Benneter SS, Summers BA, Schulz-Schaeffer WJ, et al. Mixed glioma (oligoastrocytoma) in the brain of an African hedgehog (*Atelerix albiventris*). J Comp Pathol 2014;151(4):420-4.

61. Burballa A, Martinez J, Martorell J. Splenic lymphoma with cerebellar involvement in an African hedgehog (*Atelerix Albiventris*). J Exot Pet Med 2012; 21(3):255-9.

62. McLaughlin A, Strunk A. Common emergencies in small rodents, hedgehogs and sugar gliders. Vet Clin North Am Exot Anim Pract 2016;19(2):465-99.

63. Fukuzawa R, Fukuzawa K, Abe H, et al. Acinic cell carcinoma in an African pygmy hedgehog (*Atelerix albiventris*). Vet Clin Pathol 2004;33(1):39-42.

64. Buergelt CD. Histopathologic findings in pet hedgehogs with nonneoplastic conditions. Vet Med 2002;97(9):660-5.

65. Wheler CL, Grahn BH, Pocknell AM. Unilateral proptosis and orbital cellulitis in eight African hedgehogs (*Atelerix Albiventris*). J Zoo Wildl Med 2001;32(2): 236–41.

66. Diehl KA, McKinnon JA. Eye removal surgeries in exotic pets. Vet Clin North Am Exot Anim Pract 2016;19(1):245–67.

67. Raymond J, Clarke K, Schafer K. Intestinal lymphosarcoma in captive African hedgehogs. J Wildl Dis 1998;34(4):801–6.

68. Martínez-Jiménez D, Garner B, Coutermarsh-Ott S, et al. Eosinophilic leukemia in three African pygmy hedgehogs (*Atelerix albiventris*) and validation of Luna stain. J Vet Diagn Invest 2017;29(2):217–23.

69. Ramos-Vara J, Miller M, Craft D. Intestinal plasmacytoma in an African hedgehog. J Wildl Dis 1998;34(2):377–80.

70. Snow S, Higbie C, Tully TN, et al. Multiple myeloma in an African hedgehog (*Atelerix albiventris*) based on necropsy findings. J Exot Pet Med 2019;30(1):82–4.

71. Lowden LR, Davies JL. Malignant neuroendocrine tumour (carcinoid) of the spleen in an African pygmy hedgehog (*Atelerix albiventris*). J Comp Pathol 2016;155(1):88–91.

72. Ogihara K, Itoh T, Mizuno Y, et al. Disseminated histiocytic sarcoma in an African hedgehog (*Atelerix albiventris*). J Comp Pathol 2016;155(4):361–4.

73. Heatley JJ. Cardiovascular anatomy, physiology, and disease of rodents and small exotic mammals. Vet Clin North Am Exot Anim Pract 2009;12(1):99–113.

74. Delk KW, Eshar D, Garcia E, et al. Diagnosis and treatment of congestive heart failure secondary to dilated cardiomyopathy in a hedgehog. J Small Anim Pract 2014;55(3):174–7.

75. Black PA, Marshall C, Seyfried AW, et al. Cardiac assessment of African hedgehogs (*Atelerix albiventris*). J Zoo Wildl Med 2011;42(1):49–53.

76. Fitzgerald BC, Dias S, Martorell J. Cardiovascular drugs in avian, small mammal, and reptile medicine. Vet Clin North Am Exot Anim Pract 2018;21(2): 399–442.

77. Johnson DH. Hedgehog and sugar gliders: respiratory anatomy, physiology, and disease. Vet Clin North Am Exot Anim Pract 2011;14(2):267–85.

78. Snider T, Joyner P, Clinkenbeard K. Disseminated histoplasmosis in an African pygmy hedgehog. J Am Vet Med Assoc 2008;232(1):74–6.

79. Needle DB, Selig MK, Jackson KA, et al. Fatal bronchopneumonia caused by skunk adenovirus 1 in an African pygmy hedgehog. J Vet Diagn Invest 2019; 31(1):103–6.

80. Rivera RY, Janovits EB. Oronasal squamous cell carcinoma in an African hedgehog (*Erinaceidae albiventris*). J Wildl Dis 1992;28(1):148–50.

81. Lennox AM, Miwa Y. Anatomy and disorders of the oral cavity of miscellaneous exotic companion mammals. Vet Clin North Am Exot Anim Pract 2016;19(3): 929–45.

82. Go DM, Woo SH, Lee SH, et al. Pleomorphic adenoma of the mandibular salivary gland in a captive African pygmy hedgehog (*Atelerix albiventris*). J Vet Med Sci 2019;81(2):177–81.

83. Helmer PJ. Abnormal hematologic findings in an African hedgehog (*Atelerix albiventris*) with gastrointestinal lymphosarcoma. Can Vet J 2000;41(6):489–90.

84. Clarke DE. Oral biology and disorders of chiroptera, insectivores, monotremes, and marsupials. Vet Clin North Am Exot Anim Pract 2003;6(3):523–64.

85. Martínez LS, Juan-Sallés C, Cucchi-Stefanoni K, et al. *Actinomyces naeslundii* infection in an African hedgehog (*Atelerix albiventris*) with mandibular osteomyelitis and cellulitis. Vet Rec 2005;157(15):450–1.

86. Cho HM, Choi US, Lee HB. Cytologic aspects of oral squamous cell carcinoma in a captive African hedgehog (*Atelerix albiventris*). J Vet Clin 2013;30(3):214–7.

87. Hrysyzen TM, Malmberg JL, Johnston MS. Diagnosis and clinical management of eosinophilic gastroenteritis in an African pygmy hedgehog (*Atelerix albiventris*). J Exot Pet Med 2019;30(3):88–91.

88. Spugnini EP, Lanza A, Sebasti S, et al. Electrochemotherapy palliation of an oral squamous cell carcinoma in an African hedgehog (*Atelerix albiventris*). Vet Res Forum 2018;9(4):379–81.

89. Adamovicz L, Bullen L, Saker K, et al. Use of an esophagostomy tube for management of traumatic subtotal glossectomy in an African pygmy hedgehog (*Atelerix albiventris*). J Exot Pet Med 2016;25(3):231–6.

90. Dierenfeld E. Feeding behavior and nutrition of the African pygmy hedgehog (*Atelerix albiventris*). Vet Clin North Am Exot Anim Pract 2009;12(2):335–7.

91. Sedlák K, Šmíd B, Šikulová M, et al. Papillomatosis in captive African pygmy hedgehog (Atelerix albiventris), vol. 6. Berlin: Proc of Institute for Zoo and Wildlife Research; 2005. p. 287.

92. Han JI, Lee SJ, Jang HJ, et al. Isolation of *Staphylococcus simulans* from dermatitis in a captive African pygmy hedgehog. J Zoo Wildl Med 2011;42(2):277–80.

93. Martin KK, Johnston MS. Forelimb amputation for treatment of a peripheral nerve sheath tumor in an African pygmy hedgehog. J Am Vet Med Assoc 2006;229(5):706–10.

94. Raeder L, Biron K, Schwittlick U. Peripheral nerve sheath tumour in an African pygmy hedgehog. Kleintierpraxis 2019;64(6):339–47.

95. Chung TH, Kim HJ, Choi US. Multicentric epitheliotropic T-cell lymphoma in an African hedgehog (*Atelerix albiventris*). Vet Clin Pathol 2014;43(4):601–4.

96. Finkelstein A, Hoover JP, Caudell D, et al. Cutaneous epithelioid variant hemangiosarcoma in a captive African hedgehog (*Atelerix albiventris*). J Exot Pet Med 2008;17(1):49–53.

97. Ramirez J, Chavez L, Aburto E, et al. Sebaceous gland carcinoma in an African hedgehog (*Atelerix albiventris*). Vet Mex 2008;39:91–6.

98. Kim HJ, Kim YB, Park JW, et al. Recurrent sebaceous carcinoma in an African hedgehog (*Atelerix albiventris*). J Vet Med Sci 2010;72(7):947–9.

99. Couture EL, Langlois I, Santamaria-Bouvier A, et al. Cutaneous squamous cell carcinoma in an African pygmy hedgehog *(Atelerix albiventris)*. Can Vet J 2015;56(12):1275–8.

100. Huang J, Eshar D, Andrews G, et al. Diagnostic challenge. J Exot Pet Med 2014;23(4):418–20.

101. Raymond JT, White MR, Janovitz EB. Malignant mast cell tumor in an African hedgehog (*Atelerix albiventris*). J Wildl Dis 1997;33(1):140–2.

102. Phair K, Carpenter JW, Marrow J, et al. Management of an extraskeletal osteosarcoma in an African hedgehog (*Atelerix albiventris*). J Exot Pet Med 2011;20(2):151–5.

103. Reyes-Matute A, Méndez-Bernal A, Ramos-Garduño LA. Osteosarcoma in African hedgehogs (*Atelerix albiventris*): Five cases. J Zoo Wildl Med 2017;48(2):453–60.

104. Benoit-Biancamano MO, D'Anjou MA, Girard C, et al. Rib osteoblastic osteosarcoma in an African hedgehog (*Atelerix albiventris*). J Vet Diagn Invest 2006;18(4):415–8.

105. Peauroi JR, Lowenstine LJ, Munn RJ, et al. Multicentric skeletal sarcomas associated with probable retrovirus particles in two African hedgehogs (*Atelerix albiventris*). Vet Pathol 1994;31(4):481–4.
106. Johnson DH. Emergency presentations of the exotic small mammalian herbivore trauma patient. J Exot Pet Med 2012;21(4):300–15.
107. Williams J. Orthopedic radiography in exotic animal practice. Vet Clin North Am Exot Anim Pract 2002;5(1):1–22.
108. Miwa Y, Carrasco DC. Exotic mammal orthopedics. Vet Clin North Am Exot Anim Pract 2019;22(2):175–210.
109. Helmer PJ, Lightfoot TL. Small exotic mammal orthopedics. Vet Clin North Am Exot Anim Pract 2002;5(1):169–82.
110. Johnson DH. Endoscopic intubation of exotic companion mammals. Vet Clin North Am Exot Anim Pract 2010;13(2):273–89.

End-of-Life Decisions
Palliative Care, Hospice, and Euthanasia for Exotic Animals

Angela M. Lennox, DVM, DABVP (Avian, Exotic Companion Mammal), DECZM (Small Mammal)

KEYWORDS

- Euthanasia • Hospice • Palliative care • Exotic animals

KEY POINTS

- Exotic animal veterinarians likely perform euthanasia at higher rates than traditional pet practitioners because of shortened lifespans of many exotic pets, and higher rate of husbandry-related diseases.
- Euthanasia is often technically more difficult in exotic pets because of anatomic differences and small size.
- Traditional intravenous (IV) euthanasia solution delivery techniques are generally inappropriate for conscious exotic animals.
- The ideal euthanasia technique has 2 parts: preanesthesia given by simple intramuscular (IM) or subcutaneous injection delivered using minimally stressful handling techniques, followed by delivery of IV, intraorgan, intracelomic, or IM euthanasia solutions in the completely anesthetized animal.

HOSPICE AND PALLIATIVE CARE

Interest in animal hospice and palliative care has increased. Owners are familiar with these concepts in human medicine and are more actively requesting the same for their pets, including exotic pets. Hospice is defined by the International Association for Animal Hospice and Palliative Care (IAAHPC) as "a philosophy or program of care that addresses the physical, emotional and social needs of animals in the advanced stages of a progressive, life-limiting illness or disability."[1] Palliative care is "treatment that supports or improves the quality of life for patients and caregivers by relieving suffering."[1] Because definitions and understanding of the 2 terms vary slightly, there is some degree of overlap between them.

The author has no commercial or financial conflicts of interest, or funding sources related to this article.
Avian and Exotic Animal Clinic, 9330 Waldemar Road, Indianapolis, IN 46268, USA
E-mail address: birddr@aol.com

Vet Clin Exot Anim 23 (2020) 639–649
https://doi.org/10.1016/j.cvex.2020.06.003
1094-9194/20/© 2020 Elsevier Inc. All rights reserved.

The American Animal Hospital Association (AAHA) and IAAHPC released a comprehensive document outlining end-of-life care guidelines in 2016.[1] Their Guidelines for Recommended Practices in Animal Hospice and Palliative Care are available online at: www.iaahpc.org/images/2017_IAAHPC_Animal_Hospice_and_Palliative_Care_Guidelines.pdf. IAAHPC also offers extensive training modules and certification in hospice and palliative care.

In general, end-of-life care represents significant challenges, including the ability to care simultaneously for both patient and owner. Ideal animal hospice addresses the emotional, social, and spiritual needs of the caregiver, which can be difficult for clinicians without some degree of preparation or training.

IAAHPC guidelines contain several useful tools and resources, including the principles of empathetic end-of-life communication, collaborative hospice planning between pet owners and veterinary team members, and grief and bereavement support.[1] Recommendations include providing most of the care in the pet's normal environment, when possible, and scheduling regular rechecks to evaluate and potentially modify hospice plan implementation.

The 3 components of animal hospice address the physical, social, and emotional needs of the pet.[1] Application of these principles to exotic pets poses unique challenges, often related to difficulties relating to objective measurement of pain, stress, and discomfort, and there being little evidence-based pain management. Careful evaluation of physical condition and limitations, knowledge of normal species-specific behaviors, and information on the pet's daily routine can help owners and veterinary staff design appropriate hospice care.

Physical care includes elements such as ability to provide nutrition, enhance mobility, ensure safety, and manage pain (managing pain is often the easiest of the 3). Examples of enhancing mobility can include a 3-sided litter box for patients who use them, nonslip surfaces and perches, and food and water provided on a single cage level or perch (**Fig. 1**). Ensuring safety may include lowering perches for birds, and providing a padded cage bottom to prevent injury in case of falls (**Fig. 2**).

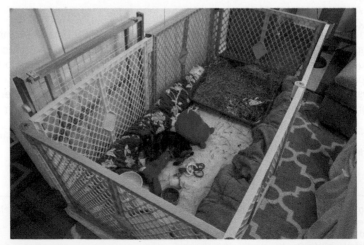

Fig. 1. At-home hospice setup for a rabbit with limited mobility. Note the 3-sided litter box, absorbent fleece pad bedding, bumpers to prevent limb entrapment in the cage sides, stuffed animal supports, and easily accessible food and water. (*Courtesy of* D. Sailer, Indianapolis, IN.)

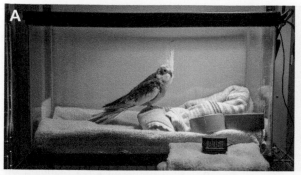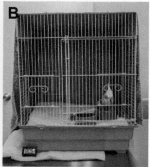

Fig. 2. At-home hospital or hospice setups for birds using an aquarium (*A*) or a cage with perches removed and a towel at the bottom (*B*). Both options allow better temperature control and prevent injuries in case of falls. Food and water are easily accessible. Note the indoor/outdoor thermometers.

Measuring and ensuring emotional well-being may present a significant challenge. Some exotic pets give few clues on emotional or social well-being, in particular many reptile and amphibian species. Birds and some exotic mammals are more social, and every attempt should be made to allow social groups to remain together. This outcome can be accomplished by housing social groups or bonded pairs side by side, or in a cage within the main cage; this allows patients in hospice to exist in a group without competing for food or other resources and risk of bullying (**Fig. 3**). Other suggestions for hospice care for exotics pets are presented in **Table 1**.

Although euthanasia is a well-accepted end-of-life option for veterinary patients, comprehensive palliative care allowing natural death at home should be considered an acceptable alternative as well. IAAHPC provides guidelines for humane natural hospice-supported death. This alternative is in sharp contrast to allowing a pet to die without euthanasia or effective palliative care, which is considered unethical and inhumane.[1]

EUTHANASIA

Euthanasia is a combination of Greek words meaning good (eu) and death (thanatos). The goal of euthanasia is to minimize pain, distress, and negative effect to the animal

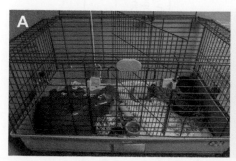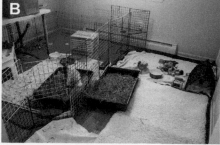

Fig. 3. (*A*) A bonded pair of guinea pigs housed in the same cage with a barrier to protect the hospice pig on the right from competition or bullying from his companion on the left. (*B*) Two geriatric angora rabbits in side-by-side cages. ([*B*] *Courtesy of* D. Sailer, Indianapolis, IN.)

Table 1
Hospice and palliative care considerations modified from components of an integrated approach to end-of-life care, American Animal Hospital Association/International Association for Animal Hospice and Palliative Care end-of-life care guidelines[1]

Considerations		Exotic Companion Mammals	Pet Birds	Reptiles
Physical care	Pain management	Evidence-based analgesia whenever possible; careful observational skills to detect inadequate analgesia (most challenging in many reptile species)		
	Hygiene	Sanitary grooming of perineum, careful removal of feces/urine	Regular removal of droppings adhered to feathers	Regular removal of feces
		Easy-access litter boxes (when applicable)		
	Nutrition	Keep food/water within easy reach, support feeding using minimal-stress techniques and species-appropriate products		
	Mobility	Solid nonskid flooring	Lower padded and easy-to-grip perches	Newspaper or paper towels
	Safety	Use single-level housing, protect from other pets	Provide low perches and padded enclosure bottom to protect in case of a fall	
Social well-being	Engagement with family and companions	Many reptiles are not social; provide privacy and limit handling	-include	-include
	Mental stimulation	Encourage accustomed activities, offer less challenging forms of enrichment		
Emotional well-being	Stress reduction	Assess stress level associated with medical care, minimize changes in routine	Limit handling	

associated with the illness.[2] Of equal importance is ensuring that the euthanasia is performed using techniques that minimize stress for the pet and the owner, who may wish to be present, and maximize comfort. For conscious exotic pets, this almost always means abandoning the traditional simple intravenous (IV) administration techniques that are commonly used in dogs and cats.

The American Veterinary Medicine Association (AVMA) has published and updated guidelines for euthanasia (*AVMA Guidelines for the Euthanasia of Animals*).[2] Although guidelines have existed since 1963, the 2013 edition greatly expanded specific species recommendations, including those for exotic pet species such as birds, reptiles, small mammals, fish, and even crustaceans and fertile eggs. This version, and the most recent 2020 version, contains a wealth of useful information on the entire process, including decision making on when to choose euthanasia.[2] Note that the guidelines encourage presedation/anesthesia before administration of euthanasia solutions for all species unless administration will not produce stress; for example, for an ill pet that is not responding to stimuli.[2]

American Veterinary Medicine Association unacceptable techniques

In general, any technique that produces stress, discomfort, or pain is unacceptable. AVMA guidelines mention several methods that should be obviously unacceptable, including hypothermia, drowning, and administration of household chemicals. Some techniques are only acceptable for operators with special training, including cervical dislocation, decapitation, and gunshot; these are generally not within the scope of discussion for common exotic pet species.

Other unacceptable techniques include intraorgan administration in conscious patients, intracelomic administration in birds (because of the presence of air sacs), and overdose of inhalant anesthetic agents in conscious patients.

Although inhalant overdose seems to be a humane alternative, time to death can be prolonged, and can produce stress. Inhaled anesthetics are considered aversive to rabbits and rodents, and produce behaviors that suggest anxiety; this may be true for other species as well.[2] Apnea may prolong the time to unconsciousness. The AVMA document on humane euthanasia cites the *US Government Principles for the Utilization and Care of Vertebrate Animals Used in Testing, Research and Training*, which states that procedures that cause pain or distress in humans should be considered likely do the same in animals as well.[3] In a study in human children 2 to 10 years old, more than 40% showed significant stress responses, some severe, to sevoflurane induction.[4,5]

Inhalant overdose is also inappropriate when owners wish to be present; not only is death prolonged but there is potential for human exposure to higher levels of inhalant agents. Although adverse effects in humans secondary to isoflurane and sevoflurane exposure are not well documented, potential effects from other volatile agents include genotoxic, hepatotoxic, and possibly teratogenic and reproductive effects. Concern for potential risk has led to the development of isoflurane and sevoflurane exposure limits in many countries.[6]

The Occupational Safety and Health Administration (OSHA) currently states: "The levels of risk for isoflurane, desflurane, and sevoflurane have not been established. Since there are limited data, occupational exposure limits for these agents have not been determined. Therefore, until more information is available, it is prudent to attempt to minimize occupational exposure to these as with all anesthetic agents."[7]

Isoflurane exposure was quantified in laboratory animal workers using direct active gas sampling and infrared spectroscopy. Results showed minimal exposure with the use of good room ventilation, ideally constructed and used anesthetic equipment (including intubation), and effective active gas scavenging.[8] Chamber or facemask administration of isoflurane for euthanasia is likely to markedly increase human exposure and should be avoided.

The AVMA guidelines state that other unacceptable methods of euthanasia include delivery of euthanasia solution via the intraosseous (IO) route in conscious patients because of the pain and stress of IO catheter placement.[2]

For reptiles, AVMA guidelines currently exclude hypothermia or freezing as a humane technique.[2] However, current research suggests that freezing of body tissues may not produce pain or anxiety.[9] Continuous and smooth decline in brain function was recorded in cane toads exposed to gradual cooling.[9]

Under consideration

Intracelomic administration of euthanasia solutions in conscious animals is an attractive option that requires little technical skill. Intracelomic administration seems effective in mammal and reptile species; however, the AVMA euthanasia guidelines indicate there is insufficient evidence on whether or not this route produces discomfort or stress.[2] For this reason, intracelomic may not be an ideal route of administration in conscious patients.

American Veterinary Medicine Association acceptable methods and acceptable with modifications

Acceptable methods of euthanasia include IV administration and administration via an IV catheter when delivery is not expected to produce stress.[2] Because this is unlikely to be the case in exotic species, deep sedation, or preferably anesthesia, is recommended before euthanasia.[2] Once the patient is unconscious, euthanasia solutions can be administered via intraorgan (when feasible), intracelomic, IV, or IO routes. The author regularly administers intramuscular (IM) euthanasia solutions in completely anesthetized exotic patients.

Overdose of injectable anesthetics administered using minimally stressful techniques is also considered an acceptable means of euthanasia.[2]

Intracardiac administration of euthanasia solutions is acceptable when venipuncture is considered humane in that species (eg, snakes).[2] Euthanasia techniques applicable to pet exotic species are presented in **Table 2**.

Anesthesia before euthanasia

For conscious exotic pets, deep sedation or complete anesthesia is ideal before euthanasia; however, administration of anesthetics can be stressful as well. In the author's experience, stress of induction is mitigated by combining high dosages of anesthetic drugs into a single syringe for simple IM injection using minimal restraint and handling techniques (**Table 3**).

Level of anesthesia is evaluated carefully before administration of euthanasia solutions. If the patient is still responsive, additional dosages are administered.

Once the animal is completely unconscious, euthanasia solutions can be administered by many routes, including IV, IO, intraorgan,[2] and even IM (in the author's personal experience). Dosages of drugs used at the author's practice for injectable anesthesia before euthanasia are listed in **Table 3**. Note that very debilitated patients may require lower dosages of anesthetics; alternatively, patients in shock or organ failure may require higher dosages and/or longer time to induction because of poor metabolism and/or distribution from the IM injection site.

Table 2
Euthanasia techniques for mammals, birds and reptiles based on recommendations from the American Veterinary Medicine Association Guidelines for the Euthanasia of Animals, 2020 Edition[2]

Recommendation	Technique
Acceptable	Intraorgan, IO, intracelomic, intramuscular[a] administration in completely unconscious animals
	Sedation and placement of an IV catheter, followed by IV administration of euthanasia solution
	Intracardiac administration in snakes
	Overdoses of injectable anesthetics in any species
Acceptable with modifications	Direct IV administration or via an IV catheter if this can be accomplished without stress (this is unlikely in conscious exotic species)
Unacceptable	Intraorgan, IO, IM administration in conscious animals
	Overdose of inhalant agents in conscious animals
	Thoracic compression in avian species
	Intracelomic administration in avian species

[a] Intramuscular administration in the unconscious animal is not addressed in the AVMA euthanasia guidelines.

Notes on less common exotic species

The AVMA guidelines list overdose of anesthetics and complete anesthesia followed by IV or intraorgan administration as acceptable methods of euthanasia for pet fish. Of interest is that flushing is listed in the guidelines as an unacceptable technique.[2] Anesthesia protocols for fish are well described. For exotic practitioners not regularly

Table 3
Agents and dosages useful for anesthesia before euthanasia in exotic pet species

Agent	Dose (mg/kg)	Comment
Xylazine	10–20	Inexpensive and effective, pain on injection is likely to be minimal
Opioids	Standard therapeutic dosages	Enhances effects of other agents, analgesia
Dexmede-tomidine	—	Very effective in high doses, but is expensive
Ketamine	10–20	Effective when combined with other agents, but produces pain on injection. Not preferred for this reason
Alfaxalone	5–20	Lower doses are highly effective when combined with other agents. Much higher (up to 10× higher) dosages required when used alone; expensive
Tiletamine-zolazepam	20	Expensive
Midazolam	1–2	Antianxiety; to enhance other agents listed above

Selected agents (usually 2–4) are combined into a single syringe and injected using low-stress minimal handling techniques.

seeing fish patients, alfaxalone is often readily available and an excellent drug for fish anesthesia.[10]

The guidelines also provide information for euthanasia of invertebrates, fetuses, and fertile eggs.[2]

Oral Administration of Euthanasia Solutions

There are anecdotal reports of administration of oral euthanasia solutions in fractious dogs. One published report on oral administration studied voluntary ingestion of euthanasia solution placed in cookie dough with flavorings in laboratory mice as a way to accomplish stress-free and handling-free euthanasia. Although mice ingested plain cookie dough readily, once pentobarbital-containing euthanasia solution was added, palatability was affected and volumes consumed were not enough to produce unconsciousness.[11] The 2020 AVMA guidelines do not recommend oral administration of euthanasia solution without further study. The author uses euthanasia solution orally in injured wildlife where handling is risky; for example, adult raccoons with neurologic signs. Solution is delivered via syringe and blunt needle through the cage bars and causes rapid deep sedation/anesthesia at approximately 1.5 mL/kg by mouth. Additional euthanasia solution is administered by injection.

CLIENT PREPARATION AND PARTICIPATION

In the author's, more owners wish to be present than not, and their presence is never discouraged. Once the decision for euthanasia is made, the veterinary staff's role is to support the decision and provide a safe space for grief.[12] Many owners have witnessed pet euthanasia in the past, and may be expecting a traditional rapid IV approach. In any case, education is important so owners understand how euthanasia will proceed in exotic species, and to expect a slower, multistep procedure. Interestingly, many clients comment that euthanasia of their exotic pet was far less stressful than for their dogs and cats, where practitioners sometimes struggled to find a vein, or the pet vocalized or twitched during euthanasia. Note that AVMA guidelines recommend sedation or anesthesia before euthanasia for all companion animals when the owners wish to be present.[2]

STAFF EDUCATION AND PREPAREDNESS

Euthanasia protocols should be firmly established and uniform for all clinicians, especially for unusual species that may not be regularly encountered. Client care aspects should be reviewed periodically and rehearsed as necessary to ensure a minimally stressful and efficient process for all. Systems for euthanasia of exotic pets in the author's practice are summarized in **Box 1**.

Accommodations for euthanasia include designated comfort rooms, buzzer/bell systems owners can use to signal when finished visiting, ability to finish financial transactions in the comfort room to ensure privacy, and even separate exits for grieving owners, and these are becoming standard in many veterinary practices. Comfort rooms can include bottled water, extra tissues and wipes, literature on grief resources, and toys or other distractions for children (**Fig. 4**).

Euthanasia of a pet is an experience of utmost emotional significance for owners, and deserves serious consideration from the moment of the decision to when the client leaves the veterinary hospital. Ensuring a reduced-stress and compassionate experience requires a solid plan with all staff members actively involved and participating.

Box 1
Summary of euthanasia procedure used at the author's practice

The owner is escorted to the comfort room to discuss end-of-life decisions and spend time with the pet, if desired

A client care team member obtains written consent, and discusses body care decisions

Final financial transactions are completed

Medical team members explain or reinforce what to expect, and ask the owners to signal with the call button when they are ready to proceed

Experienced team members administer IM anesthetics using minimally stressful techniques. The pet is briefly separated from the owner to avoid accidental needle sticks or bites at the time of injection

The level of anesthesia is periodically checked; additional anesthetic is administered if necessary

Euthanasia solution is administered intraorgan, IV, intracelomic, or IM

Death is confirmed, and the owner allowed to visit as long as is desired

The body and/or paw print are prepared for return to the owner if applicable; the owner is escorted out of the clinic after asking whether there are additional questions or requests

If cremation is selected, the body and paperwork are prepared as directed by the crematorium

Euthanasia selected in the clinic software automatically generates a reminder for a sympathy card

Cremation selected in the clinic software automatically generates a reminder to ensure procedures are followed and the ashes returned to the owners.

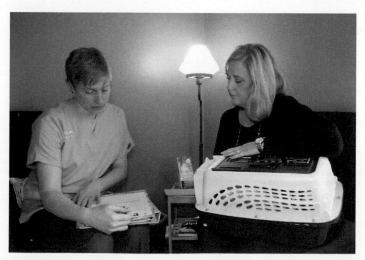

Fig. 4. An examination room repurposed as a visitation or comfort room. Paperwork, detailed explanations of the euthanasia process, and financial transactions can be accomplished in a private setting away from the traffic of a busy hospital.

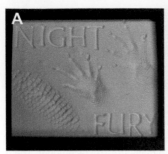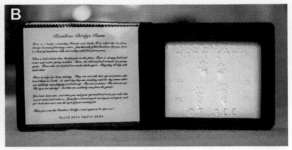

Fig. 5. No-baking clay paw print kits. Foot and tail print from a reptile (*A*) and paw prints from hamster (*B*).

Euthanasia Consent

Owner's Name:_____ Date:_____

Pet's name: _____ Species: _____

I certify that to the best of my knowledge, my pet has not bitten any person or animal within the last 10 days nor has he or

she been exposed to rabies. _____(Initial)

Aftercare Arrangements:

I request that my pet's remains be cared for in the following manner:

☐ **Private cremation**. I wish to have my pet individually cremated with ashes returned to me.

☐ **Communal cremation**. I wish to have my pet cremated with ashes scattered.

☐ **Commemorative Paw Print**. I would like a clay paw print made for my pet.

☐ **Home burial**. I would like to take my pet's remains home. (No additional charge)

☐ I would like to donate my pet's remains for educational purposes. (No additional charge)

I am the owner or authorized agent of this pet and I understand that I am responsible for all costs associated with the euthanasia and aftercare of this pet. I give the Avian and Exotic Animal Clinic full and complete authority to perform euthanasia services. Arrangements for aftercare will be as documented above. I agree to indemnify the Avian and Exotic Animal Clinic from any loss or liability.

Please sign to indicate you have read and understand the above or had the information explained to your satisfaction.

Your name (printed): _____ Client ID #: _____
Your Signature: _____ Date: _____

Avian and Exotic Animal Clinic|9330 Waldemar Rd, Indianapolis IN 46268 |www.exoticvetclinic.com

Fig. 6. Euthanasia consent form used for procedures at the author's clinic. (*Courtesy of* Avian and Exotic Animal Clinic, Indianapolis, IN.)

POSTEUTHANASIA CARE OF EXOTIC PETS

Most crematory companies provide services for exotic pets, and some set prices depending on the weight of the animal. Other services may be appropriate for exotic pets, including decorative urns, paw prints, and photographic memorials. Another attractive option is in-clinic paw print kits. These kits are easy to use and can be completed within a few minutes for the owner to take home. Creative staff members can incorporate a small feather or swatch of fur into the clay (**Fig. 5**).

For the go-home option, variably sized boxes should be available to accommodate a wide variety of exotic pet sizes. At the author's practice, donating the pet's remains for education purposes carries no additional charge. Education purposes include student/intern/resident practice for procedures such as necropsy and placement of IO catheters. Many owners find comfort in this option (**Fig. 6**).

REFERENCES

1. Bishop G, Cooney K, Cos S, et al. 2016 AAHA/IAAHPC end-of-life care guidelines. J Am Anim Hosp Assoc 2016;52(6):341–56.
2. AVMA Guidelines for the Euthanasia of Animals: 2020 Edition. Available at: www.avma.org/sites/default/files/2020-01/2020_Euthanasia_Final_1-15-20.pdf. Accessed January 22, 2020.
3. PHS Policy on Humane Care and Use of Laboratory Animals. National Institutes of Health. Available at: https://olaw.nih.gov/policies-laws/phs-policy.htm. Accessed December 21, 2019.
4. Chorney JM, Kain ZN. Behavioral analysis of children's response to induction of anesthesia. Anesth Analg 2009;109:1434–40, 145.
5. Przybylo HJ, Tarbell SE, Stevenson GW. Mask fear in children presenting for anesthesia: aversion, phobia, or both? Paediatr Anaesth 2005;15:366–70.
6. Molina Aragones JM, Ayora Ayora A, Barbara Ribalta A, et al. Occupational exposure to volatile anaesthetics: a systematic review. Occup Med 2016;66:202–7.
7. Anesthetic gases: guidelines for workplace exposure. United States Department of Labor. Available at: www.osha.gov/dts/osta/anestheticgases/#C2. Accessed November 10, 2019.
8. Johnstone K, Lau C, Whitelaw J. Evaluation of waste isoflurane gas exposure during rodent surgery in an Australian university. J Occup Environ Hyg 2017;14(12):955–64.
9. Shine R, Amiel J, Munn A, et al. Is "cooling then freezing" a humane way to kill amphibians and reptiles? Biol Open 2015;4:760–3.
10. Bugman AM, Langer PT, Hadzima E, et al. Evaluation of the anesthetic efficacy of alfaxalone in oscar fish (Astronotus ocellatus). Am J Vet Res 2016;77(3):239–44.
11. Dudley ES, Bolvin G. Evaluation of a commercially available euthanasia solution as a voluntarily ingested euthanasia agent in laboratory mice. J Am Assoc Lab Anim Sci 2018;57(1):30–4.
12. Morris P. Managing pet owner's guilt and grief in veterinary euthanasia encounters. J Cont Ethnography 2012;41(3):337–65.

Pathology of Diseases of Geriatric Exotic Mammals

Drury R. Reavill, DVM, DABVP (Avian and Reptile & Amphibian Practice), DACVP[a],*,
Denise M. Imai, DVM, PhD, DACVP[b]

KEYWORDS

- Rodents • Rabbit • Ferret • Geriatric • Neoplasia • Chronic respiratory disease
- Chronic progressive nephropathy • Atrial thrombosis

KEY POINTS

- Neoplasia is the most prevalent geriatric disease of small companion rodents, guinea pigs, rabbits, and ferrets.
- Chronic respiratory disease complex, cardiomyopathy, and chronic progressive nephropathy in aged rats.
- Atrial thrombosis with congestive heart failure in aged hamsters.
- Pododermatitis is not uncommon in older rats, mice, guinea pigs, and rabbits.
- Some infections are more common in older animals such as mycoplasma in rats, mycobacteria in ferrets, cryptococcus in ferrets, cestode cysts in rabbits, and internal and external parasites in rats and hamsters.

INTRODUCTION

Much of what we know about aging in small rodents (mice and rats) comes from studies on inbred laboratory strains[1–3] that are maintained under controlled conditions. This is also true for laboratory ferrets, rabbits, and guinea pigs.[4–6] With the interest in understanding human aging and developing interventional therapeutics to slow or reverse these aging processes, rodent, rabbit, and ferret models of aging are well defined[2,3] and the lesions of aging, both clinically significant and incidental, have been well described.[1,2,4–12] Only clinically significant and/or relatively prevalent disease processes are discussed here and include neoplastic diseases and respiratory, cardiovascular, gastrointestinal, renal, vestibular, neurologic, hepatobiliary, endocrine, musculoskeletal, and infectious diseases. The resources listed in the references

[a] ZNLabs Veterinary Diagnostics, 7647 Wachtel Way, Citrus Heights, CA 95610, USA;
[b] Comparative Pathology Laboratory, University of California, 1000 Old Davis Road, Building R1, Davis, CA 95616, USA
* Corresponding author.
E-mail address: Drury@vin.com

Vet Clin Exot Anim 23 (2020) 651–684
https://doi.org/10.1016/j.cvex.2020.06.002
1094-9194/20/© 2020 Elsevier Inc. All rights reserved.

vetexotic.theclinics.com

should be used to explore additional histopathologic lesions associated with aging in small rodents, rabbits, and ferrets, if of interest.

Relative prevalence of disease processes for mice, rats, and hamsters was based on a retrospective survey of pathology reports from the Veterinary Medical Teaching Hospital and Comparative Pathology Laboratory at the University of California, Davis. Prevalence of diseases does not directly correlate with cause-of-death assignation; for example, a rat may have multiple benign tumors but may have died of respiratory disease. The survey of rats and hamsters was collected from complete necropsy reports spanning a 20-year period, from 2000 to early 2020. The survey of mice was collected from complete necropsy reports spanning a 2-year period, from 2017 to 2018. The inclusion criteria for age varied by species; rats older than 1.5 years, mice older than 15 months, and hamsters older than 12 months were included.

The disease conditions of elderly guinea pigs, rabbit, and ferrets were collected from material in the literature, and the selected specific conditions were augmented with data from Zoo/Exotic Pathology Service (1998–2019). Guinea pigs at 3 years and rabbits and ferrets at 5 years and older were considered geriatric.

DISEASES BY ORGAN SYSTEM
Respiratory Disease

Respiratory disease was far more common in the aged rats surveyed than in the mice or hamsters (**Table 1**). Among the aged rats with respiratory disease in this retrospective survey, the most common diagnosis was chronic respiratory disease (CRD) (45 of 88 rats, 51.1%). CRD is a pneumonic complex classically considered to be initiated by an inhaled irritant (ammonia) or viral infection (Sendai virus) and promoted by infection with either or both *Mycoplasma pulmonis* and cilia-associated respiratory (CAR) bacillus.[8] In many cases, *M pulmonis* can be the primary pathogen, and murine respiratory mycoplasmosis has been used as a synonym for this respiratory disease complex.[8] The classic lesion of CRD is suppurative bronchopneumonia with bronchiectasis and abscessation. It is the bronchiectasia that gives the characteristic "cobblestone" gross appearance to the lungs, and the lobar distribution of disease is often asymmetric (**Fig. 1**). Histopathologically, respiratory mycoplasmosis incites a striking hyperplasia of the bronchial-associated lymphoid tissue. If there is a concurrent CAR bacillus infection, filamentous bacteria will be present in parallel with respiratory cilia. The prevalence of CRD in this study group is likely underrepresented as the diagnosis of bronchopneumonia—etiology (unspecified) was reported in 23 rats (26.1%) and probably represents unrecognized CRD. Pulmonic pseudotuberculosis due to *Corynebacterium kutscheri* was identified in 6 (6.8%) of the 88 rats. The gross appearance of pseudotuberculosis is distinct from CRD, manifesting as multiple foci of consolidation and necrosis (**Fig. 2**) without the asymmetric distribution or bronchiectatic appearance. The histopathologic pattern of neutrophilic inflammation with large colonies of amorphous bacteria is considered pathognomonic.[8] Bordetellosis (*Bordetella bronchiseptica*) and chronic passive pulmonary congestion (CPPC) due to cardiac insufficiency was each identified in 2 of the 88 rats (2.3%).

In the aged mice surveyed, eosinophilic crystalline pneumonia (ECP) accounted for most of the cases (5 of 6, 83.3%). ECP (alternatively called acidophilic macrophage pneumonia) can be extensive and often occurs after other pulmonary diseases (pulmonary adenomas, CPPC, and so forth).[7,10] Grossly, the pattern is interstitial to alveolar with tan to brown discoloration and failure to collapse in a regional to lobar distribution. Histologically, alveoli are filled with foamy macrophages and extracellular and intracellular sharp acicular brightly eosinophilic crystals (**Fig. 3**). A neutrophilic

Table 1
Retrospective survey of diseases in pet and laboratory rodents

Species	Total No.	Age Range	Average Age	Tumors	Respiratory Disease	Cardiomyopathy	Chronic Nephropathy	Otitis/Inner Ear Infarction	Degenerative Neurologic Disease	Dermatitis	Infectious Disease
Rats	195	1.5–4y	2.3 y	151 (77.4%)	88 (45.1%)	50 (25.6%)	62 (31.8%)	33 (16.9%)	15 (7.7%)	7 (3.6%)	82 (42.1%)
Mice[a]	79	1.3–2.3 y	1.6 y	51 (64.6%)	6 (7.6%)	32 (40.5%)	30 (40.0%)	8 (10.1%)	2 (2.5%)	4 (5.1%)	0 (0.0%)**
Hamster	23	I–2.5 y	1.4 y	16 (69.6%)	6 (26.1%)	9 (39.1%)	10 (43.5%)	0 (0%)	0 (0%)	2 (8.7%)	3 (13.0%)

[a] Three pet mice, 76 laboratory mice (strain C57BL/6J). ** 96.2% of the aged mouse population were housed in controlled specific pathogen free laboratory conditions, therefore the prevalence of infectious disease does not correlate to the companion animal population.
Data collected from the Veterinary Medical Teaching Hospital (2000-early 2020) and Comparative Pathology Laboratory (2017-2018) at the University of California, Davis.

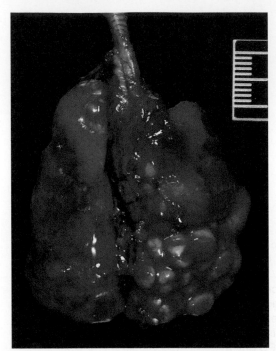

Fig. 1. Chronic respiratory disease in a rat, exhibiting the characteristic asymmetric "cobblestone" appearance caused by bronchiectatic abscessation. The causal agents include *Mycoplasma pulmonis* and CAR bacillus, with or without underlying Sendai virus infection. (*Courtesy of* C. M. Reilly, DVM, Davis, CA.)

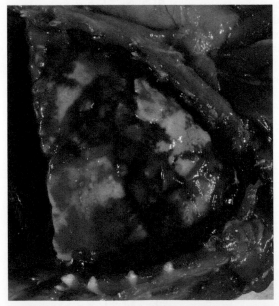

Fig. 2. Pulmonic pseudotuberculosis in a rat, caused by *Corynebacterium kutscheri*. The distribution of the tan foci of necrosis and suppurative inflammation is multifocal to coalescing. (*Courtesy of* J. Magnusson Wulcan, DVM, Davis, CA.)

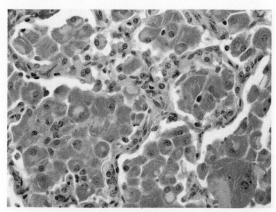

Fig. 3. Eosinophilic crystalline pneumonia in a mouse. Prevalence increases with age and with the existence of another pulmonary disease, such as a pulmonary adenoma or chronic passive congestion. Hematoxylin and eosin stain. 400x magnification.

interstitial pneumonia, smooth muscle metaplasia, and occasionally papillary intra-bronchial granulation tissue can accompany ECP. The composition of the crystals is YM1 chitinase,[7] derived from activated macrophages and is part of the systemic hya-linosis seen as an incidental finding in the respiratory, biliary, and gastric epithelium of aged mice.[7,11] CPPC due to congestive left-sided heart failure was present in 2 of the 6 mice (33.3%) with respiratory disease and occurred simultaneously with ECP in one mouse.

The most common respiratory disease in the aged hamsters was CPPC (4 of 6, 66.7%) due to heart failure. Grossly, CPPC presents with an interstitial pattern, where the lung diffusely is pale pink to tan and fails to collapse. Histologically, in CPPC, alve-olar spaces are filled with variable amounts of fluid and hemorrhage as well as foamy macrophages that contain erythrocytes or hemosiderin pigment (heart failure cells). The most common cause of CPPC in hamsters (and in mice) is left atrial thrombosis (see cardiovascular section).[9] One of 6 hamsters had gram-negative bacterial pneu-monia (16.7%), and the last hamster had interstitial pneumonia (16.7%) with features of sepsis and possibly, CPPC.

Cardiovascular Disease

Cardiovascular disease was less common in aged rats (54 of 195, 27.7%) than in mice (34 of 79, 43.0%) or hamsters (10 of 23 hamsters, 43.5%) but can affect up to 80% of the population in some rat strains.[8] Most of the cardiovascular diagnoses was cardio-myopathy (50 out of 54, 92.6%) with 25 rats having moderate-to-severe disease based on histopathologic changes in the heart and/or indicators of fulminant left-sided heart failure. Left ventricular hypertrophy (**Fig. 4**) with thickening of the ventricular wall and stenosis of the lumen was the most frequent indicator of cardiomyopathy. Infectious myocarditis (due to *Streptococcus pneumoniae*) was present in 1 of 54 (1.9%) rats. Polyarteritis nodosa (PA) was present in 1 of 54 (1.9%) aged rats. PA is characterized by chronic fibrinoid arteritis with mural dissections to saccular aneurysms, periarterial fibrosis, and luminal thrombosis. Any medium-sized artery can be affected, except in the lung.[8] Six rats (11.1%) had arteriosclerosis, a nonspecific thickening of the arterial wall.

In the aged mice, the 39 cases of cardiovascular disease were primarily cardiac. Mild to marked left ventricular hypertrophy (32 of 39, 82.1%) was the most common

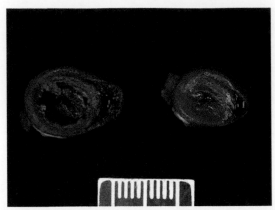

Fig. 4. Left ventricular hypertrophy in a rat. The cross-section of the affected heart (*right*) exhibits a thickened left ventricular wall and interventricular septum with collapse or stenosis of the lumen. A normal, unaffected heart on cross-section (*left*) is present for comparison.

diagnosis with a single case of dilative cardiomyopathy reported. Histopathologic changes are characterized by cardiomyocyte hypertrophy, disarray, and karyomegaly with variably mononuclear cell infiltration and fibrosis.[1,7] Left-sided congestive heart failure was documented in 2 of the 32 mice (6.3%). Chronic necrotizing arteritis (CNA), the mouse equivalent of PA, was diagnosed in 7 of 39 (17.9%). CNA in the mouse is typified by fibrinoid degeneration and necrosis of the tunica media with variable cellular inflammation, fibrosis, and luminal stenosis.[7] CNA differs from PA as it is not associated with aneurysmal weakening of the vascular wall and thus lacks the nodular component that defines PA. CNA tends to involve arteries in the head, heart, kidneys, mesentery, tongue, and urogenital tract though involvement of the gastrointestinal system and pancreas also occurs.[7,10] A single diagnosis of endocardiosis was reported, the prevalence of which is likely underrepresented, as it is difficult to consistently evaluate murine heart valves in section. Other age-related clinically significant diseases that were not reported in these mice include left auricular thrombosis.

In the aged hamsters, atrial thrombosis (**Fig. 5**) was the most common diagnosis (6 of 10, 60%) and would seem grossly as a firm mass within the left atrium/auricle. If present for some duration, the left side, and often the right, of the heart is hypertrophied. Classically, the pathogenesis of atrial thrombosis has involved renal amyloidosis[9] presumably due to loss of antithrombin III and has been thought to result in anasarca[6]; however, in this survey, none of the hamsters with atrial thrombosis had either lesion. Instead, the development of renal amyloidosis with subsequent anasarca (protein-losing nephropathy) may occur simultaneously with atrial thrombosis, as both are diseases of aging in hamsters.

Renal Disease

Chronic renal disease was similarly prevalent in these aged rats, mice, and hamsters (see **Table 1**). Unsurprisingly, chronic progressive nephropathy (CPN) was the most common diagnosis in the aged rats with renal disease (62 of 63, 98.4%). CPN is a major life-limiting disease in rats and is considered multifactorial, associated with advanced age, male sex, and high dietary protein.[3,8] Prolactin, from hormonally productive pituitary adenomas, has been associated with CPN but the association may be indirect, as both CPN and pituitary adenomas are diseases of aged rats. In this

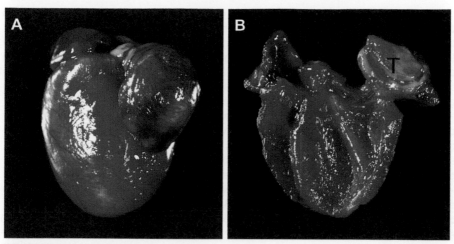

Fig. 5. Left atrial thrombosis in a hamster. (*A*) Externally, the left atrium is enlarged and firm. (*B*) On cut section, the left atrial lumen is filled with a tan lamellar thrombus (T) that is firmly adhered to the endocardial surface. (*Courtesy of* M. A. Highland, DVM, PhD, Manhattan, KS.)

retrospective survey, there was no statistically significant relationship between the 2 (Fisher's exact test, $P = .07$). The classic presentation of CPN is a light red to brown kidney with a pitted to finely cystic cortical surface (**Fig. 6**). Histologic changes are consistent with a chronic glomerulonephropathy with tubular degeneration and proteinuria. Glomerular changes include mesangial thickening, basement membrane thickening, synechiae formation, and sclerosis. Tubular changes include degeneration and cystic dilation with protein casts. Interstitial fibrosis and lymphoplasmacytic inflammation can accompany the glomerulonephropathy.[8] One rat out of the 63 had chronic cystitis with ureteral obstruction (1.6%).

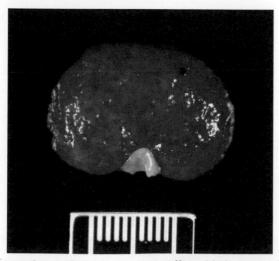

Fig. 6. Chronic progressive nephropathy in a rat. Affected kidneys are shrunken and pale tan to brown with a pitted to cystic surface. The small cortical cysts represented dilated, ectatic tubules.

Chronic nephropathy (CN) in the aged mouse resembles CPN in the rat and was diagnosed in 30 out of 36 mice (83.3%) with renal disease. The gross and histopathologic appearance of CN in the mouse is similar to the rat but is thought to begin with tubular changes and progress to membranoproliferative glomerulonephritis.[7,10,12] In certain cases, glomerular mesangial or basement membrane thickening can be so strikingly amorphous that it can be confused with amyloidosis[1] and is called hyaline glomerulopathy (HG) (**Fig. 7**).[13] In general, HG is more common than glomerular amyloidosis in the mouse (0 cases of amyloidosis in this survey), and there are histopathologic features that can distinguish between the 2 diseases. In HG, in contrast to glomerular amyloidosis, mesangial deposits can asymmetrically affect the glomerulus, and glassy thrombi can be present in glomerular capillaries. In glomerular amyloidosis, deposits are uniformly distributed within the glomerulus, and amyloid is present in at least 1 other tissue.[13] The prevalence of CN in C57BL/6 mice can approach 100% in aged colonies.[10] Pyelonephritis (3 of 36, 8.3%), unilateral hydronephrosis (2 of 36, 5.6%), and urolithiasis (1 of 36, 2.8%) comprise the remaining diagnoses of renal disease in the aged mice surveyed. Another common age-related renal disease not observed in this population includes obstructive uropathy due to retrograde ejaculation (mouse urologic syndrome).[7,10,11]

Renal disease was identified in 11 of 23 (47.8%) aged hamsters, with chronic nephropathy similarly being the most common diagnosis (10 of 11, 90.9%). The last hamster of the group had chronic pyelonephritis. Renal amyloidosis was not identified in any of the hamsters in this survey but is a classic age-related disease of hamsters.[9]

Special Senses

Disorders of the special senses (ears and eyes) were observed in the rats and mice surveyed but was not reported in the hamsters. Otitis media and interna (33 of 40, 82.5%) was the most common diagnoses and cataracts was the second and only other diagnosis (11 of 40, 27.5%). Four rats had both otitis and cataracts. Mycoplasmosis was confirmed in the ear or lungs of 12 (36.4%) of the rats with otitis. In the aged mice, labyrinthine infarction due to chronic necrotizing arteritis (6 of 10, 60%) was the

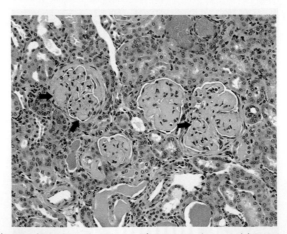

Fig. 7. Hyaline glomerulopathy in a mouse. The mesangium and basement membranes of the glomeruli are thickened by hyaline amorphous material. Capillary thrombosis, characterized by round to oval aggregates of the hyaline material (*arrows*) within capillaries, is a diagnostic feature that can be used to differentiate this entity from amyloidosis. Hematoxylin and eosin stain. 200x magnification.

most common diagnosis, followed by otitis media (2 of 10, 20%) and cataracts (2 of 10, 20%). CNA is incidental unless luminal stenosis or occlusion results in local tissue infarction, as in the ear.[10] One other age-related ocular condition of mice that was not diagnosed in this retrospective survey is ulcerative keratitis due to lacrimal gland atrophy and suboptimal tear film quality or quantity (keratoconjunctivitis sicca).[10]

Neurologic Disease

Neurologic disease was present in 20 rats (10.3%), 2 mice (2.5%), and no hamsters. In the rats, the majority (15 out of 20, 75%) had degenerative myelopathy/radiculoneuropathy, a syndrome of demyelination and axonal loss in the white matter of the spinal cord and spinal nerve roots.[8] The syndrome starts caudally, in the lumbar spinal cord and cauda equina, and manifests as posterior paresis or paralysis. Luxol fast blue can effectively highlight the extent of myelin loss as it progresses rostrally. Five of the 20 rats (25%) had a presumed bacterial meningoencephalitis or cerebellar abscess. The 2 mice identified to have neurologic disease both had compressive myelopathies subsequent to intervertebral disc degeneration (IVDD) and intraspinal canal protrusion/extrusion. IVDD is not unique to the mouse but also recognized as an age-related and life-limiting disease in rats.[8,11] IVDD, especially in the mouse, is easiest to assess histopathologically in longitudinal sections through the decalcified vertebral column. Spinal cord is best evaluated if left in situ for evaluation together with the vertebral column.

Integumentary Disease

Nononcologic integumentary diseases was identified in 3% to 9% (see **Table 1**) of the aged rat, mouse, and hamster population. In the rats, 7 of 7 (100%) diagnoses were for ulcerative pododermatitis. The cause is likely a combination of husbandry conditions, obesity in ad libitum–fed pets, and decreased grooming with general debilitation.[11] In the mice, ulcerative dermatitis (3 of 4, 75%) and pododermatitis (1 of 4, 25%) is a common disease attributed to many causes, from trichotillomania to a primary follicular dystrophy, and are often exacerbated by opportunistic staphylococcal infection.[7,10] In the hamsters, 2 cases of atrophic and fibrotic dermatopathies of unknown cause, although potentially paraneoplastic, were reported.

Infectious Disease

Infectious agents were primarily identified in the pet rats surveyed and less so in the hamsters. As the mice were laboratory animals raised in controlled conditions under stringent health surveillance, the lack of infectious disease agents was an expected finding. In the rats, agents of CRD (*Mycoplasma* sp. and CAR bacillus) were the most commonly reported (45 of 82, 54.9%). Pneumocystis sp. was identified in 2 of 82 rats (%). Fourteen rats had metazoan endoparasites (cestodes, nematodes) and 8 had arthropod ectoparasites (lice, mites). In the hamsters, demodicosis, pinworm infestation, and giardiasis was each diagnosed once, in 1 hamster.

Neoplastic Disease

The prevalence of neoplastic disease in the aged rats, mice, and hamsters ranges between 64.6% and 77.4%. Among the aged rats, 151 out of 195 rats had tumors and a total of 214 tumors were diagnosed. Based on clinical presentation (**Box 1**), subcutaneous masses were most frequently identified (56 of 195 rats, 28.7%), of which 3 had multiple types of subcutaneous tumors. The next most common were intracranial tumors in rats that presented with neurologic signs (49 of 195, 25.1%). Conversely, the most prevalent tumor diagnosis was pituitary adenoma (19.2%) (**Fig. 8**) followed by

---

Box 1
Retrospective survey of common neoplastic diseases in 196 older pet rats (1.5 years) by clinical presentation (124 tumors)

Diagnoses (No./No in category)

Subcutaneous mass
  Mammary fibroadenoma (36/59)
  Mammary carcinoma/adenocarcinoma (7/59)
  Mammary adenoma/cystadenoma (5/59)
  Subcutaneous fibroma (4/59)

Intracranial mass/Neurologic signs
  Pituitary adenoma (41/49)
  Pituitary carcinoma (2/49)
  Granular cell tumor (2/49)

Head/Neck/Oral mass
  Squamous cell carcinoma, facial, buccal, glossal, or laryngeal (10/20)
  Osteosarcoma, mandibular, or cranial (3/20)

Intrathoracic mass/Respiratory signs
  Lymphoma, pulmonary, mediastinal, or hilar (11/18)[a]

Disseminated masses
  T-cell lymphoma/leukemia (7/14)
  Non-B-cell, non-T-cell lymphoma (3/14)
  LGL lymphoma/leukemia (3/14)
  Myeloid leukemia (1/14)

Endocrine signs
  Islet cell adenoma/insulinoma (4/14)
  Pheochromocytoma (3/14)[b]
  Adrenocortical adenoma (3/14)

Reproductive mass
  Ovarian granulosa theca cell tumor (2/13)
  Endometrial adenocarcinoma (2/13)
  Uterine stromal tumor (2/13)
  Uterine leiomyosarcoma (2/13)

Hepatosplenic/Abdominal mass
  Histiocytic sarcoma (6/10)[c]

Axial/appendicular mass
  Fore/hindlimb soft tissue sarcoma (3/7)[d]

Abbreviation: LGL, large granular lymphocytic. [a] Eight were typed as B-cell origin by immunohistochemistry. [b] Two were bilateral. [c] Three were suspected. [d] Includes peripheral nerve sheath tumor and fibrosarcoma.

Data collected from the Veterinary Medical Teaching Hospital, University of California, Davis (2000-early 2020).

---

mammary fibroadenoma (16.8%) (**Fig. 9**). The actual prevalence of mammary fibroadenomas may be slightly higher, as a few rats had a history of subcutaneous tumor removal without a biopsy diagnosis. An association between mammary fibroadenomas and prolactin-producing pituitary adenomas has been suggested[5] but remains unsubstantiated. In this retrospective survey, there was no statistically significant relationship between the 2 (Fisher's exact test, $P = .3706$). Mammary fibroadenoma occurred with pituitary adenoma/carcinoma in 20 out of 43 rats (46.5%) with pituitary tumors. Mammary fibroadenoma occurred without the presence of a pituitary tumor in 13 out of 36 rats (36.1%) with mammary fibroadenoma.

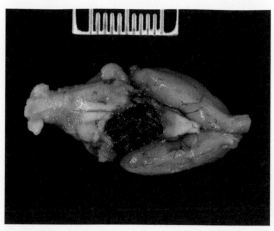

Fig. 8. Pituitary adenoma in a rat.

Other common tumor diagnoses in the aged rats included orofacial squamous cell carcinoma (**Fig. 10**), intrathoracic lymphoma, disseminated lymphoma/leukemia, and intraabdominal histiocytic sarcoma (see **Box 1**). Less common diagnoses (1–2 cases) presenting as subcutaneous masses included lymph node hemangioma, preputial squamous cell carcinoma, mammary myoepithelioma, peripheral nerve sheath tumor, fibrosarcoma, and lipoma. Less common diagnoses presenting as intracranial disease included a cerebral lymphoma and astrocytoma. Less common diagnoses presenting as masses in the head, neck, and oral region include an anaplastic sarcoma, soft tissue sarcoma, Harderian gland adenoma, B-cell lymphoma, and lip papilloma. Less common diagnoses presenting as intrathoracic masses included thymoma, mediastinal hibernoma, pulmonary carcinoma, fibrosarcoma, and osteosarcoma. Less common diagnoses presenting as endocrine disease included thyroid/c cell adenoma, thyroid carcinoma, and parathyroid adenoma. Less common diagnoses presenting with reproductive disease included a prostatic carcinoma, Leydig cell tumor, uterine histiocytic sarcoma, cervical leiomyoma, and uterine myxoma. Less common diagnoses presenting as a hepatosplenic or intraabdominal mass included an exocrine

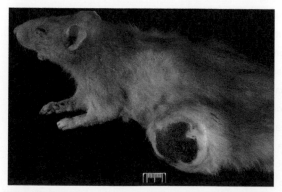

Fig. 9. Mammary fibroadenoma in a rat. The red to brown staining around the eyes and on the forelimbs is chromodacryorrhea. Other features of age-associated debilitation include scruffiness of the hair coat and possible ectoparasitism.

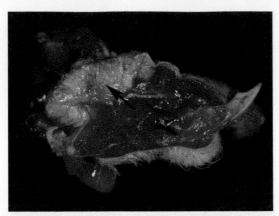

Fig. 10. Glossal squamous cell carcinoma in a rat. The mandible is transected along midline with the tongue in situ. The black arrow indicates the tumor.

pancreatic carcinoma, splenic stromal sarcoma, splenic lymphoma, and biliary adenoma. Less common diagnoses presenting as an axial or appendicular mass included a hindlimb leiomyosarcoma, hindlimb hemangiosarcoma, malignant chordoma, and femoral osteosarcoma. Less common diagnoses presenting as an integumentary mass included a trichofolliculoma, dermal fibroma, sebaceous cystadenoma, dermal lipoma, and squamous cell carcinoma. Less common diagnoses presenting with gastrointestinal disease included a pyloric adenocarcinoma, intestinal lymphoma, colonic sarcoma, and colonic polyp.

In mice, the strain of mouse dictates the prevalence of and types of tumors that occur with age.[1,3,7,10–12] As these mice surveyed are mostly C57BL/6, the strain-specific tumor prevalence (**Box 2**) is not directly translatable to pet mice but can be used as a diagnostic guide. In this mouse strain, hematopoietic neoplasms are known

---

Box 2
Retrospective survey of common neoplastic diseases in 79 aged mice (15 months+) (68 total tumors)

Diagnoses (No.)

Histiocytic sarcoma (15)

Lymphoma/Pleomorphic lymphoma (9)

Pulmonary adenoma (6)

Harderian gland adenoma (6)

Hemangiosarcoma, subcutaneous (4)

Cutaneous papilloma, lip, or muzzle (3)

Pituitary adenoma (3)

Keratoacanthoma (2)

Pulmonary carcinoma (2)

Hepatic adenoma (2)

Data collected from the Veterinary Medical Teaching Hospital (2000-early 2020) and Comparative Pathology Laboratory (2017-20188) at the University of California, Davis.

to be very common.[10] As expected, the most common tumors in this study were histiocytic sarcoma (17 out of 51 mice with tumors, 33.3%) and lymphoma (9 of 51, 17.6%). Histiocytic sarcoma typically presents as abdominal distention due to hepatosplenomegaly (**Fig. 11**) with variable hematogenous dissemination[14] but can be localized to an axial or appendicular region (2 of the 17 cases, 11.8%). Expected gross findings with histiocytic sarcoma are an enlarged, light red to brown, variably mottled liver and spleen. The reticular pattern can be enhanced or there can be multiple pale tan foci that are nodular (representing neoplastic cellular infiltration) or depressed (representing necrosis). The histopathologic pattern of histiocytic sarcoma in the mouse is distinct; the neoplasm begins in the liver, in a sinusoid-dependent pattern that is initially more expansile than obliterative. The neoplastic histiocytes are small, oval to angular to plump spindle-shaped with modest amounts of cytoplasm and small but pleomorphic and folded nuclei.[14] Multinucleated cells are often present, and a characteristic associated lesion is renal tubular epithelial hyalinosis.[7,10,14] Immunohistochemical markers for macrophage antigens can be used to confirm the diagnosis. Most of the lymphomas were consistent with T-cell lymphoma (8 of 9 tumors), and 1 case was diagnosed as a follicular (pleomorphic) lymphoma. Most lymphomas in C57BL/6 mice are composed of moderately sized (lymphoblastic) cells with a characteristic "starry sky" appearance and aggressively disseminate to multiple sites.[14] Follicular (pleomorphic) lymphoma arises in the splenic follicles, is composed of a mixture of small and large blastic follicular center cells, and can include bi- or multinucleated cells.[12,14] These histopathologic features can be confused with histiocytic sarcoma but is differentiated from histiocytic sarcoma by the primary splenic follicular involvement and dissemination to lymphoid structures.[14] Pulmonary adenomas are typically incidental but can be clinically significant (causing dyspnea) if large enough or if associated with ECP. Harderian gland adenomas typically present with unilateral exophthalmos[10] or facial asymmetry.[7] Other common mouse tumors that are not

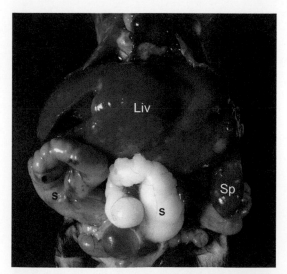

Fig. 11. Histiocytic sarcoma in a mouse. The liver (Liv) and spleen (Sp) are markedly enlarged and mottled red to pale tan with nodular aggregates scattered throughout. In this aged male mouse, the seminal vesicles (s) are also enlarged and the right seminal vesicle is orange to pink in color. Distention and color change in the seminal vesicles is a common incidental finding in aged male mice.

represented in this study due to strain-bias include mammary or salivary gland myoepitheliomas, rhabdomyosarcomas, and osteosarcomas.[7]

In the aged hamsters, 23 neoplastic diseases were diagnosed in 16 hamsters, of which 5 hamsters had multiple types of tumors. Lymphoma was the most prevalent tumor type (5 of 23, 21.7%). Three of the cases were disseminated T-cell lymphomas and 2 were epitheliotropic T-cell lymphomas. Both types of tumors are recognized as spontaneous tumors of hamsters and not necessarily associated with infection by hamster polyomavirus.[9] Epitheliotropic T-cell lymphoma presents characteristically with patchy alopecia with erythroderma and ulceration (**Fig. 12**). Diagnostic findings are characterized by monomorphic neoplastic lymphocytes aggregating within the epidermis (Pautrier microabscesses). Adrenocortical tumors (an adenoma and a carcinoma) were identified in 2 hamsters, and biliary cystadenomas were identified in 2 hamsters. Other tumor diagnoses included sebaceous adenoma, hepatoma, hemangiosarcoma, plasmacytoma, mucinous carcinoma, ovarian cystadenoma, pituitary adenoma, renal adenoma and carcinoma, scrotal sarcoma, splenic sarcoma, uterine leiomyoma, and dermal histiocytic sarcoma.

Other Clinically Significant Changes Associated with Aging

Foreign-body periodontitis,[7,10,11] caused by the lodging of hair shafts in the gingival sulcus with subsequent reactive inflammation and bony resorption, is an age-related disease in mice that can result in dental attrition and inanition. Seminal vesicular dilation is age related in male mice and although impressive and possibly causing space-occupying disease, is largely an incidental finding.[7,10,11] In hamsters, polycystic liver disease[9] can result in hepatic dysfunction and visceral compression.

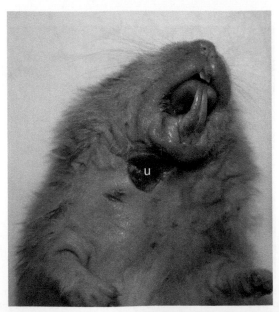

Fig. 12. Epitheliotropic T-cell lymphoma (mycosis fungoides) in a hamster. The typical presentation, depicted here, is alopecia with thickening and ulceration (u) of the skin. (*Courtesy of* K. D. Watson, DVM, PhD, DACVP, Davis, CA.)

GUINEA PIGS

Guinea pigs are vocal, interactive pets that will live up to 5 to 7 years. They are generally considered senior around 3 to 5 years. A select number of diseases specific to guinea pigs are described based on submissions to Zoo/Exotic Pathology Service from 1998 to late 2019. Additional entities are selected based on recent publications that add more information about the disease/lesion.

DISEASES BY ORGAN SYSTEM
Integumentary Disease

Older males (boars) can accumulate large amounts of waxy, malodorous, sebaceous material in the skin of the perianal region.[15] This material is often mistaken for a fecal impaction (**Fig. 13**). The circumanal region contains a large number of perineal sebaceous glands that in the male are used for scent marking. The sebaceous glands are testosterone dependent; females have much smaller glands and in castrated males the gland atrophy and are infiltrated with fat.[16] Intact adult males also have a deeper perineal sac than females and castrated males so the secretions tend to accumulate in the folds of the circumanal and genital region.[16]

Musculoskeletal Disease

Guinea pigs are prone to pododermatitis, and this is a common finding in older animals.[17] The lesion is a painful ulcerative and/or erosive inflammation of the footpads that can become severe enough to affect the phalanges as an osteolysis (**Fig. 14**). Secondary bacterial involvement, usually Staphylococcus aureus, can result in septicemia.[18] Typically the animals are overconditioned and housed on wire floors or on

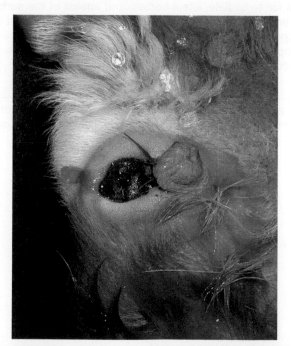

Fig. 13. Male guinea pig with accumulation of brown to black, malodorous sebaceous material around the perineum.

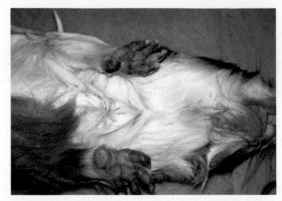

Fig. 14. Mild to moderate pododermatitis with ulceration in guinea pig. Compare with the foot in **Fig. 16.**

abrasive bedding.[18] Overweight animals may not move around enough resulting in them sitting for long periods of time on contaminated bedding with feces and urine.[19]

Reproductive Disease

Ovarian cysts are very common reproductive tract lesion, and the incidence increases with advancing age.[20] The primary cyst is a cystic rete ovarii, and these are commonly bilateral (**Fig. 15**). The rete ovarii is considered to be the remnant of an embryonic structure in adult animals. These cysts are usually located in the hilus of the ovary or are limited to the mesovarium adjacent to the hilus. Cysts can also arise from Graafian follicles that fail to ovulate, luteal bodies, and infolds of the surface epithelium; however, these are rare in guinea pigs. A common associated lesion is bilateral non-pruritic flank alopecia, which is suspected to be hormonally influenced although rete ovarii are not documented to produce sex hormones.[20] One guinea pig report with a confirmed follicular ovarian cyst had elevated estrogen levels.[21]

Renal Disease

Renal disease is a common finding in older guinea pigs. The lesions of chronic fibrosing nephritis, interstitial nephritis, pyelonephritis, and renal cysts have been

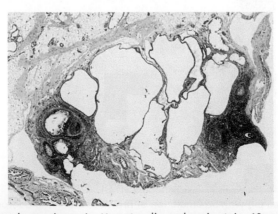

Fig. 15. Cystic ovary in a guinea pig. Hematoxylin and eosin stain. 10x magnification.

reported.[22,23] In inflammatory lesions the kidneys may be irregular grossly, and in pyelonephritis the ureters may be dilated. Chronic nephrosclerosis (fibrosing interstitial nephritis/nephrosis) is renal scarring of undetermined cause primarily due to the chronic nature of the lesion. It may be the result of vascular disease, infection, or immune-mediated disease. Grossly the renal cortex is irregularly pitted and histologically there is interstitial fibrosis, variable glomerulosclerosis, tubular dilatation, and variable mononuclear inflammation. Most cases of acquired renal cysts are associated with chronic renal disease.

Infectious Disease

Cervical lymphadenitis, one differential diagnosis for thyroid tumors, is commonly associated with *Caviibacter abscessus* (previously known as *Streptococcus zooepidemicus*).[24,25] Although this is not necessarily a lesion of older guinea pigs, it is an important differential for both thyroid lesions and lymphoma. The infection generally results in a chronic suppurative lesion, which frequently involves the cervical lymph nodes (**Figs. 16** and **17**). It can become septicemic. In young animals it tends to progress to a severe respiratory infection (fibrinopurulent pleuritis, pericarditis, and bronchopneumonia) that has a high mortality and morbidity.[26]

Neoplastic Disease

A review of neoplastic diseases diagnosed at Zoo/Exotic Pathology Service is tabulated (**Box 3**). The most common tumors in geriatric guinea pigs (5 years or greater) were mammary gland adenocarcinomas/carcinomas, lipomas, trichofolliculomas, and thyroid gland carcinomas.

Thyroid tumors are a common tumor in guinea pigs (median age 4.3 years, range 2.5–6 years).[27] The typical presentation is of a palpable mass on the ventral neck with progressive weight loss. The differential based on physical examination includes cervical lymphadenitis and lymphoma. Aspiration cytology is an easy, diagnostic method to obtain a quick answer as to the cause of cervical swellings.[28] The clinical

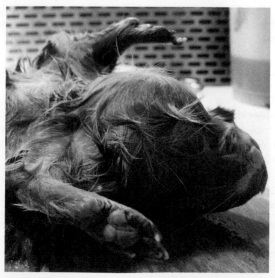

Fig. 16. A ventral cervical swelling in a guinea pig. This is similar in appearance as thyroid lesions and lymphoma.

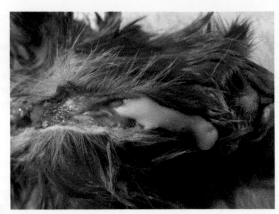

Fig. 17. The swelling has been opened to demonstrate the pus of cervical lymphadenitis in this older guinea pig.

signs in functional tumors are typical for most mammals: weight loss, increased activity, and tachycardia due to cardiomegaly. The tumors have been macrofollicular thyroid adenomas, thyroid cystadenoma, papillary thyroid adenoma, follicular thyroid carcinoma, follicular-compact thyroid carcinoma, small-cell thyroid carcinoma, and an ectopic thyroid carcinoma.[27,29] Some of the tumors may develop foci of osseous metaplasia, which may be identified by radiology (**Fig. 18**).[27,29] In one study all neoplasms were positive for thyroid transcription factor 1 and thyroglobulin but negative for parathyroid hormone and calcitonin.[27]

In guinea pigs, mammary tumors occur with equal frequency in female and male animals.[30] The age range is reported from 3 to 7.5 years.[30] The tumor types encompass papillary cystadenomas, adenomas, papillary adenocarcinoma, tubulopapillary carcinomas, adenocarcinoma, and mixed mammary.[30,31] Bilateral tumors frequently occur; however, they have a low potential for metastases. The lung is the common site for the rare metastases.[31] From one study it seems most tumors are arising from the mammary ducts, and these are positive for alpha-estrogen and progesterone receptors suggesting hormonal influence on tumor formation.[30]

Rabbit

A rabbit is considered older or senior from the age of 4 to 5 years.[32,33] The maximum age ranges from 8 to 13 years for domestic rabbits.[33,34] Many of the diseases in rabbits are similar to other elderly mammals and only a select number of diseases specific to rabbits are described based on submissions to Zoo/Exotic Pathology Service from 1998 to late 2019. Additional entities are selected based on recent publications that add more information about the disease/lesion.

DISEASES BY ORGAN SYSTEM
Cardiovascular Disease

Aging New Zealand rabbits are commonly used as models of cardiac disease in humans.[35,36] With aging there is an incorporation of fat cells and connective tissue (fibrosis) in ventricular tissue and atrioventricular nodes that affects conduction time resulting in arrhythmias.[35] Myocardial fibrosis is one of the consequences of aging, and this affects the myocardial stiffness that impairs cardiac function. The causes for myocardial disease include hypovitaminosis E,[37] bacterial infection (salmonella,

Box 3
Retrospective survey of common neoplastic diseases in 341 older adult pet guinea pigs (5.0 years+) by clinical presentation (223 total tumors)

Diagnoses (No./No. in category)

Subcutaneous mass
  Mammary gland adenocarcinoma/carcinoma (45/145)
  Lipoma (27/145)
  Trichofolliculoma (25/145)
  Mammary gland adenoma/cystadenoma (9/145)
  Fibrolipoma (6/145)
  Liposarcoma (5/145)
  Soft tissue sarcoma (4/145)
  Myxosarcoma (4/145)
  Neurofibrosarcoma (3/145)
  Epitheliotropic lymphosarcoma (3/145)
  Squamous cell carcinoma (3/145)
  Carcinoma, site not provided (2/145)
  Extraskeletal osteosarcoma (2/145)
  Lymphoma (1/145)
  Malignant melanoma (1/145)
  Fibrosarcoma (1/145)
  Hemangioma (1/145)
  Myxoma (1/145)
  Trichoepithelioma (1/145)
  Leiomyosarcoma (1/145)

Head/Neck/Oral mass
  Lymphoma, lymph nodes (2/4)
  Odontogenic tumor (1/4)
  Sarcoma, poorly differentiated (1/4)

Intrathoracic mass/Respiratory signs
  Pulmonary adenoma (5/5)

Disseminated masses
  Lymphoma (8/8)

Endocrine signs
  Thyroid gland carcinoma (10/12)
  Thyroid gland adenoma (2/12)

Reproductive mass
  Leiomyoma/fibroleiomyoma, uterus (6/18)
  Endometrial adenocarcinoma/carcinoma, uterus (4/18)
  Carcinoma, ovary (2/18)
  Leiomyosarcoma, uterus (2/18)
  Seminoma, testicle (1/18)
  Endometrial adenoma, uterus (1/18)
  Squamous cell carcinoma, uterus (1/18)
  Deciduoma, uterus (1/18)

Hepatosplenic/Abdominal mass
  Sarcoma (autolyzed or poorly differentiated) (5/24)
  Hepatic biliary cystadenoma (4/24)
  Leiomyosarcoma, intestine (3/24)
  Neurofibrosarcoma, stomach/intestine (3/24)
  Hemangiosarcoma, spleen (2/24)
  Hemangiosarcoma, stomach (1/24)
  Hemangioma, spleen (1/24)
  Lymphoma, spleen (1/24)
  Leiomyoma, cecum (1/24)
  Leiomyoma, site not determined (1/24)

Hepatic biliary carcinoma (1/24)
Fibrosarcoma, site not determined (1/24)

Urinary mass
Lymphoma (urinary bladder) (1/2)
Soft tissue sarcoma (urinary bladder) (1/2)

Skeletal mass
Osteosarcoma, limb (2/5)
Osteoma, vertebral column (1/5)
Fibrosarcoma, limb (1/5)
Carcinoma, limb (1/5)

pasteurella),[38] and encephalitozoonosis.[39,40] Rabbits that are fed a hyperlipemic diet are models for myocardial fibrosis and coronary atherosclerosis in man.[36]

Digestive Tract Diseases

Dental disease in older rabbits includes malocclusion typically from the loss of an opposing tooth, tooth root abnormalities, and abscesses.[41] There are many complete reviews and books written about rodent and rabbit dental disease, and the reader is referred to the published literature.

Chronic abscesses especially associated with the oral cavity and dental diseases are common in older rabbits.[41] These pyogranulomatous abscesses can invade into the mandibular or maxillary bones. Even with complete surgical removal and appropriate antibiotics these abscesses frequently recur.[41] Abscesses can occur in many organs when the causative bacteria go septic.[41]

The mucosal recto-anal papilloma is an uncommonly reported lesion in rabbits. It has been described primarily in older rabbits and demonstrated to be nonviral in origin.[42,43] There is no sex predilection, and the age range is 1 to 11 years with a median age of 4.8 years.[42] These are usually well-differentiated cauliflower-like growths that arise from the anorectal junction, and they are reported to be benign (**Fig. 19**). Complete surgical removal is recommended although too little information is available to determine if these undergo neoplastic transformation in other mammalian species.

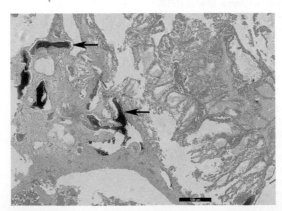

Fig. 18. Guinea pig thyroid gland carcinoma with osseous metaplasia (*arrows*). Hematoxylin and eosin stain. 2x magnification.

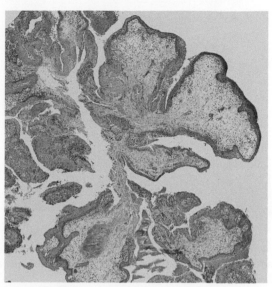

Fig. 19. Rabbit rectoanal papilloma. Hematoxylin and eosin stain. 2x magnification.

Integumentary Disease

Sebaceous adenitis is widely reported in rabbits. To date, this has been primarily in older animals. It presents as a nonpruritic scaling dermatitis with patchy to coalescing areas of alopecia. Biopsy is usually opted, as these will have little response to many treatments, including antimicrobials and antiinflammatories. On histology, there will be several changes that include hyperkeratosis, follicular interface dermatitis, and reduction in the numbers of sebaceous glands with possible association of lymphocytic infiltrations. Perifollicular to diffuse dermal fibrosis is also noted. The differentials should include dermatophytes as well as ectoparasitic infections. It seems that there is an increasing association between these lesions in adult rabbits and thymomas.[19]

A common nontumorous skin mass is the collagen nevi (collagenous hamartoma). The median age is 6 years. This nodular, raised, firm skin lesion has been described primarily on males. In some animals these may be solitary masses and in others, multiple nodules may develop. The common locations are on the abdomen and thorax.[44] The lesions are of haphazardly arranged collagen bundles thickening in the middermis **(Fig. 20)**.

Musculoskeletal Disease

Pododermatitis, commonly known as sore hocks, has a complex cause. This is commonly identified in older overconditioned adults. Poor sanitation, inappropriate caging such as wire-bottom cages, and bedding materials will contribute to this disease resulting in a lack of mobility.[34] Coarse bedding materials with poor liquid and ammonia binding such as straw, wood shavings, or course bark mulch are associated with lesion development.[45] These lesions develop on the plantar aspect of the metatarsal bones and are usually circumscribed ulcerative foci that may be associated with granulation tissue. Early in the lesions, there may be a purulent exudate. Staphylococcus species is the most frequent isolate from these lesions.[41]

Aging rabbits can develop degenerative spinal disease. In one study the spondylotic vertebral lesions were present in rabbits as early as 2 years. The lesions first develop in

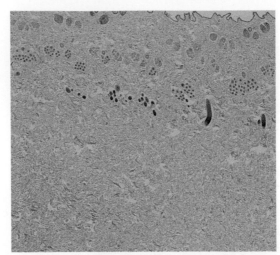

Fig. 20. Rabbit collagenous hamartoma thickening the skin in males. Hematoxylin and eosin stain. 2x magnification.

the cervicothoracic region and then the lumbar spine. The study did not evaluate the findings with clinical signs.[32] Osteoarthritis of the lumbosacral areas and hindlimbs have been noted to affect normal behavior of aging rabbits. It is not typical for the lesions to result in signs of pain or discomfort.[33]

Reproductive Disease

Endometrial hyperplasia, frequently cystic, is a common finding in rabbits.[46,47] The mean age is 4.5 years to 5.2 years,[47] which is younger than rabbits that develop uterine tumors (mean age 6.1 years).[46,47] Endometrial adenocarcinoma is the most common neoplastic lesion.[47] Frequently both conditions may be present; however, there is no documented evidence that hyperplasia progresses to a neoplastic lesion.[47,48] The development of abnormal proliferative lesions in the endometrium is under hormonal influence.[49] The ovaries of mature rabbits generally support multiple maturing follicles and corpora lutea that suggests the uterine tissue is exposed to both estrogens and progesterones continuously.[48]

Respiratory Disease

Respiratory lesions in aging rabbits are uncommonly described. Spontaneous pulmonary emphysema has been recognized in older rabbits. It was found to have minimal clinical significance and no relationship with overdistension of alveoli during ventilation.[50] One review associates the development of the lesion with atrophy of pulmonary tissue.[51]

Renal Disease

As with many mammals, aged rabbits can develop chronic renal disease (**Fig. 21**). Depending on the severity of the lesions, there may be associated metastatic mineralization of the soft tissues, particularly of the aorta. It is believed that many cases may be a lesion of chronic or previous infections of *Encephalitozoon cuniculi*.[33] A recent review of urinary tract disease covers chronic lesions as well as common neoplasms of the urinary tract.[52]

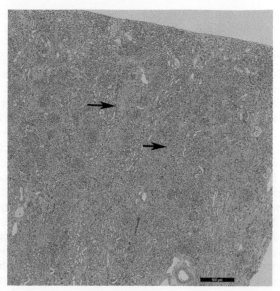

Fig. 21. Histology of chronic interstitial fibrosing nephritis in a rabbit. Arrows point to bands of fibrosis through the cortex. Hematoxylin and eosin stain. 2x magnification.

Infectious Disease

Cysticercosis is the infection of a host by the eggs of a parasitic tapeworm whose larval form creates cysts in various tissues of the body. Rabbits and hares are often the intermediate host for many cestodes, usually *Taenia multiceps*, *Taenia pisiformis*, and *Taenia serialis*, whose primary host are canids and other carnivores.[53,54] It is more commonly reported in wild rabbits and hares and rarely in domestic rabbits.[55,56] Infection rates in domestic pet rabbits are unknown but are assumed to be comparably low. Published cases of cysticercosis in pet and other caged rabbits include 2 laboratory animals that were believed to be infected via contaminated hay, but other cases do not report possible means of infection.[57,58] The parasitic cysts can be found on the liver surface, peritoneal, diaphragmatic and intestinal serosa, and in subcuticular tissues (**Fig. 22**).[58,59] These are reported to be more commonly identified in older female

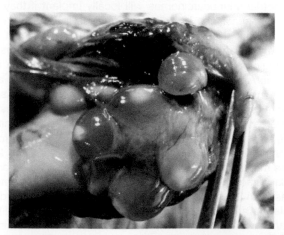

Fig. 22. Cestode cysts proliferating on the serosa of the stomach in a rabbit.

rabbits,[59] although one author (DRR) has cases evenly divided between the sexes. The age range from one author (DRR) is 1 to 9 years with a medium of 4.1 years.

Neoplastic Disease

Although tumor development increases with age, only a few tumors will be discussed. More comprehensive reviews of rabbit tumors are published.[60,61]

The reported age range for mammary gland tumor development is 8 months to 14 years; the mean age is between 4.9 and 5.5 years.[62–65] It seems that most of the invasive cancer cases develop through a stepwise progression from noninvasive forms. For many, the mammary gland starts with simple cysts or lobar hyperplasia, to benign intracystic tubulopapillary tumors, and finally to carcinomas with possible metastasis.[62–64] Both benign and malignant mammary gland lesions can occur together.[63,64] Most of the tumors reported are carcinomas and/or adenocarcinomas.[63–65] From one study both cranial and caudal glands are equally affected.[65] Unlike in human medicine, there is no standardization of tumor classification for rabbits, which complicates developing prognostic factors. The primary option for therapy is surgical removal.[66] Nearly all reported tumors are in females or neutered females and most are carcinomas.[66] These carcinomas are often negative for estrogen and progesterone receptors. This suggests the tumor growth is independent to exposure and/or progesterone. Therapy aimed at these receptors will unlikely be beneficial for most rabbits.[63] Secretory activity is commonly recognized on histology (lipid droplets in tumor cells), which can suggest prolactin influence on tumor development.[66] Tumor recurrence has been reported with matrix-producing carcinomas and adenocarcinomas.[64] Metastasis are difficult to determine in studies involving pet rabbits, as many were not evaluated further after death although vascular invasion is noted in some malignancies.[65] The metastatic sites include regional lymph nodes, kidneys, lungs, liver, pancreas, adrenal glands, ovary, and bone marrow, and rarely the eye (uvea).[61,67] In one study, 29% of the pet rabbits with mammary tumors had concurrent uterine carcinomas.[64]

Uterine tumors are the most common lesion found in the reproductive tract of female rabbits.[46] From a study with full necropsies, metastasis from endometrial adenocarcinomas was found in 44.2% of the rabbits, with the lung being the most common site.[46] Other sites include pleura and mediastinum, peritoneum and omentum, liver, kidney, ovaries, diaphragm, spleen, lymph nodes, brain, bone marrow, and urinary bladder.[47] Endometrial adenocarcinomas will locally implant if they invade through the uterine wall. The tumor can be found as masses in both uterine horns.[47] The mean age was 6.2 years.[46] Uterine adenocarcinomas are the most common tumor with lesser numbers of adenomas, leiomyosarcomas, leiomyomas, hemangiosarcoma, and hemangioma.[46] Endometrial adenocarcinomas can be subdivided into papillary and tubular/solid, which have some differences in how aggressive they invade through the myometrium. They also differ in hormonal expression. Most papillary adenocarcinomas are both estrogen receptor-a (ER) and progesterone receptor (PR) negative, whereas the more aggressive tubular/solid adenocarcinomas are positive for ER-a, PR, or both.[48] This could suggest additional therapies for hormone sensitive tumors.[48] Survival after ovariohysterectomy (OVH) was 22 to 27 months from one study. Unless metastasis can be identified, OVH should be recommended.[47]

Rabbit testicular tumors typically occur in elderly males. In a review the age range for all tumors was from 2 years to 12 years.[68] As described in sporadic case reports, 8 tumors were bilateral and 2 were metastatic in this review.[68] Most of the tumors were diagnosed as granular cell tumors (GCT), with a fewer number of seminomas, and Sertoli cell tumors.[68,69] Granular cell tumors have been recently better characterized and most tumors originally diagnosed as interstitial cell tumors have been reclassified as GCTs.[69] The age range for GCT is 2 to 11 years with a median of 7.3 years. Surgical removal carries a good prognosis.

Trichoblastomas, which are tumors arising from basal-type cells, are one of the most common skin tumors and typically occur in older rabbits (median age 5–7 years).[44,70] In general, trichoblastomas are solitary, well-circumscribed intradermal masses. The common sites of tumor occurrence are the neck, head, axilla, thorax, flank, and hindlimb.[44,70] The malignant form is very uncommon.[70]

FERRET

The lifespan of ferrets is reported to be 8 to 10 years in European reports. In North America, the average age is reported to be 5 to 7 years of age; many veterinarians consider 3 years of age as old.[71,72] The diseases and lesions commonly associated with aging include neoplastic disease as well as changes in vision, musculoskeletal degeneration, oral disease, cardiomyopathy, renal disease, and nonspecific gastrointestinal lesions. Long-term anorexia, particularly in older animals, and secondary to any other disease conditions can lead to hepatic lipidosis, a very common finding.[71]

DISEASES BY ORGAN SYSTEM
Cardiovascular Disease

Both dilated and hypertrophic cardiomyopathies have been recognized. Valvular diseases are less common, and heartworm disease is reported in areas with exposure to the disease agents. Dilated cardiomyopathy is the most common heart lesion. Changes in cardiac function are typically recognized antemortem using electrocardiograms, ultrasound, radiographs, and CT in order to make the definitive diagnosis. Gross evaluation will also confirm generalized changes to the heart, including dilated and hypertrophic hearts, as well as identification of lesions on the heart valves, and the presence of heartworm within the chambers. Histologic evaluation can add in additional information such as evidence of fibrosis indicating damage to the heart or any possible inflammatory lesion and less likely identification of disease agents that may be present.[71]

Digestive Tract Diseases

As with many mammals, aging ferrets can also develop dental calculi and not uncommonly, fractured canines.[73] Tooth fractures can occur with fighting and abnormal wear from chewing on hard surfaces.[74] Extruded canine teeth are also a common oral lesion in older ferrets.[75] With the development of dental calculi, it is not uncommon to see gingivitis. Untreated and progressive gingivitis can lead to periodontal disease, which can contribute to tooth mobility and loss.[73] Dental caries and tooth resorption seem to be very rare in ferrets, although diet may be an influencing factor.[75] Although rare, similar to domestic dogs and cats, ferrets have been reported to develop oronasal fistulae.[71,74]

Gastrointestinal diseases are fairly common in older ferrets, with trichobezoars, gastric ulcers, epizootic catarrhal enteritis, and inflammatory bowel disease (IBD) as the most commonly reported causes. Gastrointestinal foreign bodies are typically recognized in younger ferrets, with the exception of trichobezoars. From one study the age of the animals ranged from 22 to 59 months, with a mean of 43.7 months compared with an age mean of 22.4 months with other foreign bodies (sponges and rubber items). Trichobezoar formation may be due to excessive grooming or the accumulation of fur around a previously ingested nidus of material.[76]

IBD is a common, idiopathic, chronic disorder of the gastrointestinal tract in ferrets older than 1 year. The mean age for IBD is reported at 4.1 years[77] and 3 years.[78] The disease presents with nonspecific clinical signs but related to the digestive tract: nausea, anorexia, weight loss, diarrhea, melena, and rectal prolapse. The definitive diagnosis requires full-thickness intestinal biopsies, in order to differentiate from intestinal lymphoma.[78] A histologic grading scheme that correlates with the severity of the clinical signs has been developed in order to provide more consistent evaluation for prognosis.[78] Histologically, IBD is characterized by blunting of the intestinal villi and by a lymphoplasmacytic inflammatory infiltrate of the mucosa. The cause of IBD is yet undetermined. The treatment of IBD generally consists of suppression of the inflammatory response with azathioprine or corticosteroids.

Spleen

Nonspecific splenic enlargement is fairly common in older ferrets (**Fig. 23**). This can be secondary to any number of disease conditions, including tumors, myeloid hyperplasia, and chronic congestion such as from heart disease as well as nodular hyperplasia. Extramedullary hematopoiesis is a very common cause for enlargement. The initiating factor for this particular proliferation is unknown in ferrets.[71]

Renal Disease

It seems aging ferrets, particularly those older than 4 years, will have varying degrees of chronic interstitial nephritis. This is typically a progressive change that may result in dysfunction and possibly failure. Renal cysts are also not uncommon, which can occur secondary to the lesions of interstitial nephritis with obstructive lesions of renal ducts and/or renal tubules. There is a form of inherited polycystic disease with multiple cysts identified both in the kidneys as well as occasionally in the liver of young ferrets.[52]

Infectious Disease

Mycobacterial infections are reported in pet ferrets, although uncommon. It is a more significant disease with *Mycobacterium bovis* in feral ferrets of New Zealand.[79] As chronic infections, these are typically diagnosed in older ferrets (3–6 years). The microbes have been of a variety of species: *Mycobacterium xenopi* (probable aquarium origin), *Mycobacterium genavense*, *Mycobacterium avium* subsp *hominissuis*, and *Mycobacterium celatum*.[80–86] The clinical signs are diverse and depends on the major

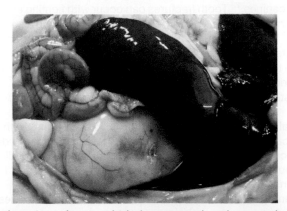

Fig. 23. Large spleen in a ferret, which is congested and supporting extramedullary hematopoiesis.

organ system involved. Progressive weight loss is a consistent finding. Concurrent diseases or immunosuppression are not always present.[81,82,84] The histologic lesions are of granulomatous inflammation with macrophages and multinucleated giant cells with cytoplasmic acid-fast bacteria. Treatment has been attempted in some cases; however, the infection recurred in most cases after discontinuation of therapy.[82,83,85,86]

Cryptococcus infections are uncommon in ferrets but as mycobacteria, can be chronic infections more commonly identified in older ferrets.[87] The clinical signs are related to the organ system involved and include lymphadenopathy, blindness, rhinitis, dermatitis, pneumonia, and meningitis.[88] *Cryptococcus gattii* seems to be more virulent than *Cryptococcus neoformans* and will cause infection in immune-competent hosts. The infection in ferrets is generally protracted as opposed to the rapid dissemination to the central nervous system reported in other species.[88] Cytology of the lesions reveals mixed inflammation (multinucleated giant cells, macrophages, and neutrophils) and generally large numbers of yeast with the characteristic morphology of a thick, nonstaining capsule. The source of the infection is environmental and typically associated with Eucalyptus trees.[87,88]

Neoplastic Disease

Although tumor development increases with age, only a few tumors are discussed. More comprehensive reviews of ferret tumors are published covering more details.[60,89,90]

Adrenal disease is a common hyperplastic to neoplastic lesion in aging ferrets (**Fig. 24**). In reports the mean age is 4.4 years and the median age is 4.5 years.[90] Tumors of the adrenal gland are reported to be the most common tumor in ferrets.[90] The tumors are primarily cortical carcinomas and adenomas.[90] Uncommonly, pheochromocytomas and neuroblastomas arise in the medulla.[90] Mesenchymal tumors are also reported: leiomyosarcomas, leiomyomas, and spindle cell sarcomas.[90] It has been shown that there is correlation with the age of neutering to the development of the very common proliferative and/or neoplastic adrenal cortical tumor of ferrets.[91] The study was comparing ferrets in Europe, which are neutered much later than ferrets in North America. European ferrets developed adrenal gland lesions at an older age. The lesion does seem to be related to the act of neutering of the animal and removal of those reproductive hormones. The sex of the animal had no association with

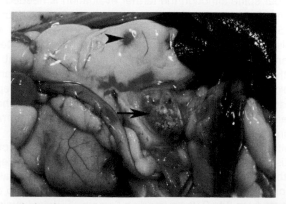

Fig. 24. Right adrenal gland tumor (*arrow*) and kidney buried in perirenal fat (*arrow* head) in a ferret.

development of adrenal gland lesions.[91] In adrenal gland disease, it is not uncommon for one or more of the sex steroids to elevate: estradiol, 17-hydroxyprogesterone, or androstenedione. These hormones can lead to vulvar enlargement in female, squamous metaplasia of the prostate in male ferrets and commonly progressive, symmetric alopecia. The disease currently is less commonly identified, as surgical removal of the adrenal glands has fallen out of favor compared with medical treatment with leuprolide acetate (Lupron). This is a gonadotropin-releasing hormone analogue. Lupron does result in reduction of clinical signs but will not affect the size of affected adrenal glands. With the advent of the common use of Lupron, adrenal gland tumors that are surgically removed seem to occur in older ferrets and the tumors are more aggressive (personal observation DRR).

Pancreatic islet cell tumors (insulinoma or pancreatic islet B-cell tumor) are also a very common endocrine tumor in middle-aged to older ferrets and in some studies the most common tumor in ferrets.[92] In studies the age range is 2 years to 8 years (median 5 years).[90] Some reports suggest there is a male sex predilection.[72] Islet cell tumors are most frequently beta cell tumors and are functional.[92] These cells produce insulin, which can result in hypoglycemia. The lesions range from hyperplasia to adenomas and adenocarcinomas. The tumors have a high recurrence rate but are slow to metastasize. The common sites of metastases are liver, spleen, and lymph nodes.[72]

Most of the pancreatic tumors arise from the isles of Langerhans. Fewer numbers of exocrine tumors have been described. Exocrine pancreatic carcinomas are aggressive tumors of older ferrets.[93] The clinical signs are nonspecific, usually weight loss and the development of ascites. The tumor typically widely metastasizes into organs (liver, lung, intestines) and/or seeds the abdomen as carcinomatosis.[93]

Lymphoma is a common tumor identified in older animals. In studies the mean age ranges from 5.2 years to 6.8 years.[77,94] There is an apparent difference in the tumor type based on the age of the ferret. Juvenile ferrets typically have more high-grade lymphomas. Most of the lymphomas in adults have a slower progression and a more chronic pattern than the juvenile form. Multicentric and gastrointestinal forms are the more common presentations.[95] Multicentric forms will involve superficial lymph nodes, as well as the mesenteric lymph nodes, spleen, and liver.[94,95] Gastrointestinal lymphoma develops nodular to diffuse lesions of the intestines, particularly the small intestines, and the mesenteric lymph nodes.[95] Gastric lymphoma in ferrets is reported to be associated with *Helicobacter mustelae* infection (a B-cell lymphoma).[96] Skeletal lymphoma has been described as aggressive lytic osseous lesions usually involving the lumbar spine although the further evaluation is needed for this uncommon presentation.[94,97,98] Immunohistochemistry seems to be a factor in prognosis with survival of 5 months with T-cell lymphomas and 8.4 months with B-cell lymphoma.[99] The clinical signs will vary depending on the organ system affected but does include generalized weakness, depression, anorexia, weight loss, vomiting, and changes in the gastrointestinal functions.[71,94] Nonregenerative anemia is a common finding on blood analysis.[94,95,99] Hypercalcemia has also been reported as a paraneoplastic syndrome in ferrets. In these ferrets the parathyroid hormone–related protein levels were elevated with suppressed intact parathyroid hormone as characterized for humoral hypercalcemia of malignancy.[98]

Cutaneous epitheliotropic lymphoma typically presents as areas of a progressive, pruritic dermatitis. The neoplastic lymphocytes infiltrate into the epidermis, outer root sheaths of the follicles, and adnexa. These are T-cell lymphomas.[100]

Mast cell tumors are a common cutaneous tumor. These tend to arise in middle-aged to older ferrets from 2 to 9 years (median 5 years). Surgical excision is generally curable and these tumors do not metastasize. Multiple tumors can develop.[101] The tumors are small, round to plaquelike masses frequently with surface crusting. They develop commonly on the extremities and the trunk. Histologically they are sheets of infiltrative mast cells associated with eosinophils. The mast cell cytoplasmic granules stain poorly with hematoxylin and eosin stains.

A less common cutaneous tumor is a dermal leiomyosarcomas. The age range is 3- to 6-year-old ferrets. They appear as single cutaneous nodules. These tumors are discrete masses originating from smooth muscle of the arrector pili, with no site preference. Most are malignant tumors although with completer removal they do not appear to recur or metastasize. Poorly differentiated tumors may require immunohistochemistry to differentiate from fibrosarcomas and malignant peripheral nerve sheath tumors. In one study there was a slight sex predilection in males.[102] From the database of ZEPS, this was also noted with 22 males (neutered and intact) and 8 females (neutered and intact) with a median age 5.3 years (range 4–7 years).

DISCLOSURE

The authors have no commercial or financial conflicts of interest nor any funding sources.

REFERENCES

1. Brayton CF, Treuting PM, Ward JM. Pathobiology of aging mice and GEM: Background strains and experimental design. Vet Pathol 2012;49:85–105.
2. Sundberg JP, Berndt A, Sundberg BA, et al. The mouse as a model for understanding the chronic diseases of aging: the histopathologic basis of aging in inbred mice. Pathobiol Aging Age Relat Dis 2011;1:7179.
3. Carter CS, Richardson A, Huffman DM, et al. Bring back the rat! J Gerontol A Biol Sci Med Sci 2020;75:405–15.
4. Fox JG, Marini RP. Research and applications. In: Biology and diseases of the ferret. 3rd edition. Ames (IA): Wiley-Blackwell; 2014. p. 627–795.
5. Barthold SW, Griffey SM, Percy DH. Rabbit. In: Pathology of laboratory rodents and rabbits. 4th edition. Ames (IA): Wiley-Blackwell; 2016. p. 253–323.
6. Barthold SW, Griffey SM, Percy DH. Guinea pig. In: Pathology of laboratory rodents and rabbits. 4th edition. Ames (IA): Wiley-Blackwell; 2016. p. 213–52.
7. Barthold SW, Griffey SM, Percy DH. Mouse. In: Pathology of laboratory rodents and rabbits. 4th edition. Ames (IA): Wiley-Blackwell; 2016. p. 91–117.
8. Barthold SW, Griffey SM, Percy DH. Rat. In: Pathology of laboratory rodents and rabbits. 4th edition. Ames (IA): Wiley-Blackwell; 2016. p. 134–71.
9. Barthold SW, Griffey SM, Percy DH. Hamster. In: Pathology of laboratory rodents and rabbits. 4th edition. Ames (IA): Wiley-Blackwell; 2016. p. 194–8.
10. Pettan-Brewer C, Treuting PM. Practical pathology of aging mice. Pathobiol Aging Age Relat Dis 2011;1:7202.
11. Snyder JM, Ward JM, Treuting PM. Cause-of-Death analysis in rodent aging studies. Vet Pathol 2016;53:233–43.
12. Haines DC, Chattopadhyay S, Ward JM. Pathology of aging B6:129 mice. Toxicol Pathol 2001;29:653–61.
13. Hoane JS, Johnson CL, Morrison JP, et al. Comparison of renal amyloid and hyaline glomerulopathy in B6C3F1 mice: An NTP retrospective study. Toxicol Pathol 2016;44:687–704.
14. Frith CH, Ward JM, Harleman JH, et al. Hematopoietic system. In: Mohr U, editor. International classification of rodent tumors; the mouse. Berlin: Springer; 2001. p. 417–49.

15. Nakamura C. Reproduction and Reproductive Disorders in Guinea Pigs. Exot DVM 2000;2(2):11–7.

16. Iburg TM, Arnbjerg J, Ruelokke ML. Gender differences in the anatomy of the perineal glands in Guinea pigs and the effect of castration. Anat Histol Embryol 2013;42(1):65–71.

17. White SD, Guzman DS-M, Paul-Murphy J, et al. Skin diseases in companion guinea pigs (Cavia porcellus): a retrospective study of 293 cases seen at the Veterinary Medical Teaching Hospital, University of California at Davis (1990-2015). Vet Dermatol 2016;27(5):395-e100.

18. Brown C, Donnelly TM. Treatment of pododermatitis in the guinea pig. Lab Anim (NY) 2008;37(4):156–7.

19. Ritzman TK. Management of integumentary lesions in the emergent exotic companion mammal patient. In proceedings ABVP. October 11-14, 2018, Tampa Florida.

20. Bertram CA, Müller K, Klopfleisch R. Genital Tract Pathology in Female Pet Guinea Pigs (Cavia porcellus): a Retrospective Study of 655 Post-mortem and 64 Biopsy Cases. J Comp Pathol 2018;165:13–22.

21. Kohutova S, Paninarova M, Skoric M, et al. Cystic endometrial hyperplasia and bacterial endometritis associated with an intrauterine foreign body in a guinea pig with ovarian cystic disease. J Exot Pet Med 2017;27:44–5.

22. Steblay RW, Rudofsky U. Spontaneous renal lesions and glomerular deposits of IgG and complement in guinea pigs. J Immunol 1997;107:1192–6.

23. Takeda T, Grollman A. Spontaneously occurring renal disease in the guinea pig. Am J Pathol 1970;60:103–18.

24. Bemis DA, Johnson BH, Bryant MJ, et al. Isolation and identification of Cavibacter abscessus from cervical abscesses in a series of pet guinea pigs (Cavia porcellus). J Vet Diagn Invest 2016;28(6):763–9.

25. LaRegina MC, Wightman SR. Thyroid papillary adenoma in a guinea pig with signs of cervical lymphadenitis. J Am Vet Med Assoc 1979;175(9):969–71.

26. Schoeb TR. Respiratory diseases of rodents. Vet Clin North Am Exot Anim Pract 2000;3(2):481–96.

27. Gibbons PM, Garner MM, Kiupel M. Morphological and immunohistochemical characterization of spontaneous thyroid gland neoplasms in guinea pigs (Cavia porcellus). Vet Pathol 2013;2013(50):334–42.

28. Barrios-Arpi LM, Morales-Cauti SM. Cytomorphological characterization of lymphadenopathies in guinea pigs: study of 31 clinical cases. J Exot Pet Med 2020;32:1–5.

29. Kondo H, Koizumi I, Yamamoto N, et al. Thyroid Adenoma and Ectopic Thyroid Carcinoma in a Guinea Pig (Cavia porcellus). Comp Med 2018;68(3):212–4.

30. Andrews EJ. Mammary neoplasia in the guinea pig (Cavia porcellus). Cornell Vet 1976;66:82–96.

31. Suárez-Bonnet A, de las Mulas JM, Millán MY, et al. Morphological and immunohistochemical characterization of spontaneous mammary gland tumors in the guinea pig (Cavia porcellus). Vet Pathol 2010;47(2):298–305.

32. Green PW, Fox RR, Sokoloff L. Spontaneous degenerative spinal disease in the laboratory rabbit. J Orthop Res 1984;2(2):161–8.

33. Benato L. How to deal with geriatric rabbits. British Small Animal Veterinary Congress 2017.

34. Fox RR. The Rabbit (Oryctolagus cuniculus) and research on aging,. Exp Aging Res 1980;6(3):235–48.

35. Gottwald M, Gottwald E, Dhein S. Age-related electrophysiological and histological changes in rabbit hearts: age-related changes in electrophysiology. Int J Cardiol 1997;62(2):97–106.

36. Orlandi A, Francesconi A, Marcellini M, et al. Role of ageing and coronary atherosclerosis in the development of cardiac fibrosis in the rabbit. Cardiovasc Res 2004;64(3):544–52.

37. Yamini B, Stein. S Abortion, stillbirth, neonatal death, and nutritional myodegeneration in a rabbit breeding colony. J Am Vet Med Assoc 1989;194(4):561–2.

38. Tomlinson CW, Dhalla NS. Alterations in myocardial function during bacterial infective cardiomyopathy. Am J Cardiol 1976;37(3):373–81.

39. Cox JC, Hamilton RC, Attwood HD. An investigation of the route and progression of Encephalitozoon cuniculi infection in adult rabbits. J Protozool 1979; 26(2):260–5.

40. Leipig M, Matiasek K, Rinder H, et al. Value of histopathology, immunohistochemistry, and real-time polymerase chain reaction in the confirmatory diagnosis of Encephalitozoon cuniculi infection in rabbits. J Vet Diagn Invest 2013; 25(1):16–26.

41. Rosenthal KL. How to Manage the Geriatric Rabbit. Atlantic Coast Veterinary Conference 2001.

42. Marcucci L, Reavill D. Rectoanal Papillomas in Rabbits: A Retrospective Review. Association of Exotic Mammal Veterinarians Conference 2014 Proceedings.

43. Meredith A. Anorectal papilloma. In: Harcourt-Brown F, Chitty J, editors. Manual of rabbit surgery, dentistry and imaging. 1st edition. Quedgeley (United Kingdom): Gloucester British Small Animal Veterinary Association; 2013. p. 254–6.

44. von Bomhard W, Goldschmidt MH, Shofer FS, et al. Cutaneous neoplasms in pet rabbits: a retrospective study. Vet Pathol 2007;44(5):579–88.

45. Wolf P, Speers R, Cappai MG. Influence of different types of bedding material on the prevalence of pododermatitis in rabbits. Res Vet Sci 2020;129:1–5.

46. Bertram CA, Müller K, Klopfleisch R. Genital Tract Pathology in Female Pet Rabbits (Oryctolagus cuniculus): a Retrospective Study of 854 Necropsy Examinations and 152 Biopsy Samples. J Comp Pathol 2018;164:17–26.

47. Walter B, Poth T, Böhmer E, et al. Uterine disorders in 59 rabbits. Vet Rec 2010; 166(8):230–3.

48. Asakawa MG, Goldschmidt MH, Une Y, et al. The immunohistochemical evaluation of estrogen receptor-alpha and progesterone receptors of normal, hyperplastic, and neoplastic endometrium in 88 pet rabbits. Vet Pathol 2008;45(2): 217–25.

49. Silverberg SG, Kurman RJ. Tumors of the uterine corpus and gestational trophoblastic disease. In: Atlas of tumor pathology, 3rd series, fascicle 3, pp. 15–89. Washinton, DC: American Registry of Pathology; 1992.

50. Cooper TK, Griffith JW, Chroneos ZC, et al. Spontaneous Lung Lesions in Aging Laboratory Rabbits (Oryctolagus cuniculus). Vet Pathol 2017;54(1):178–87.

51. Strawbridge HTG. Chronic pulmonary emphysema (an experimental study): II. Spontaneous Pulmonary Emphysema in Rabbits. Am J Pathol 1960;37(3): 309–31.

52. Reavill DR, Lennox AM. Disease Overview Of The Urinary Tract In Exotic Companion Mammals (ECM) And Tips On Clinical Management. Vet Clin North Am Exot Anim Pract 2020;23:169–93.

53. Ratliff C, Mursa A, Sladky K. Parasitic cestode cyst in the subcutaneous facial tissues of a rabbit (Octyrolagus cuniculus) (Diagnostic challenge). J Exot Pet Med 2019;31:117–9.
54. Arias-Hernández D, Flores-Pérez FI, Domínguez-Roldan R, et al. Influence of the interaction between cysticercosis and obesity on rabbit behavior and productive parameters. Vet Parasitol 2019;276:1–8.
55. Brittain PC, Voth DR. Parasites of the Black-Tailed Jackrabbit in North Central Colorado. J Wildl Dis 1975;(11):269–71.
56. Boag B, Lello J, Fenton A, et al. Patterns of parasite aggregation in the wild European rabbit (Oryctolagus cuniculus). Int J Parasitol 2001;31:1421–8.
57. Owiny JR. Cystocercosis in Laboratory Rabbits. J Am Assoc Lab Anim Sci 2001; 40(2):45–8.
58. Maas AK, Reavill DR, Schmidt R, et al. Cysticercosis in domestic pet rabbits (Oryctolagus cuniculus domesticus). Proc Assoc Exotic Mammal Veterinarians, Oakland, CA, October 23, 2012. p. 74.
59. Espinosa J, Ferreras MC, Benavides J, et al. Causes of Mortality and Disease in Rabbits and Hares: A Retrospective Study. Animals (Basel) 2020;10(1):1–17.
60. Kanfer S, Reavill DR. Cutaneous neoplasia in ferrets, rabbits, and Guinea pigs. Vet Clin North Am Exot Anim Pract 2013;16(3):579–98.
61. Heatley JJ, Smith AN. Spontaneous neoplasms of lagomorphs. Vet Clin North Am Exot Anim Pract 2004;7:561–77.
62. Greene HSN. Familial mammary tumors in the rabbit: I. Clinical history. J Exp Med 1939;70:147–58.
63. Degner S, Schoon H-A, Laik-Schandelmaier C, et al. Estrogen Receptor-α and Progesterone Receptor Expression in Mammary Proliferative Lesions of Female Pet Rabbits. Vet Pathol 2018;55(6):838–48.
64. Schöniger S, Horn LC, Schoon H-A. Tumors and tumor-like lesions in the mammary gland of 24 pet rabbits: a histomorphological and immunohistochemical characterization. Vet Pathol 2014;51(3):569–80.
65. Baum B, Hewicker-Trautwein M. Classification and Epidemiology of Mammary Tumours in Pet Rabbits (Oryctolagus cuniculus). J Comp Pathol 2015;152(4): 291–8.
66. Schöniger S, Degner S, Jasani B, et al. A Review on Mammary Tumors in Rabbits: Translation of Pathology into Medical Care. Animals (Basel) 2019; 9(10):762.
67. Eördögh R, Szikszai P, Fuchs-Baumgartinger A, et al. Bilateral uveal metastasis due to a mammary carcinoma in a rabbit: a case report. J Exot Pet Med 2019; 29:123–7.
68. Reavill D. Testicular tumors of rabbits: a survey. In: Proceedings from the International Conference on Avian, Herpetological, and Exotic Mammal Medicine. Paris, France, April 18–25, 2015. p. 452.
69. Webb JK, Reavill DR, Garner MM, et al. Characterization Of Testicular Granular Cell Tumors In Domestic Rabbits (Oryctolagus Cuniculus). J Exot Pet Med 2019; 29:159–65.
70. Kok MK, Chambers JK, Ushio N, et al. Histopathological and Immunohistochemical Study of Trichoblastoma in the Rabbit. J Comp Pathol 2017; 157(2–3):126–35.
71. Hoppes SM. The senior ferret (Mustela putorius furo). Vet Clin North Am Exot Anim Pract 2010;13(1):107–22.
72. Bakthavatchalu V, Muthupalani S, Marini RP, et al. Endocrinopathy and Aging in Ferrets. Vet Pathol 2016;53(2):349–65.

73. Nemec A, Zadravec M, Račnik J. Oral and dental diseases in a population of domestic ferrets (Mustela putorius furo). J Small Anim Pract 2016;57(10):553–60.
74. Thas I, Cohen-Solal NA. Acquired oronasal fistula in a domestic ferret (Mustela putorius furo). J Exot Pet Med 2014;23(4):409–14.
75. Eroshin VV, Reiter AM, Rosenthal K, et al. Oral examination results in rescued ferrets: clinical findings. J Vet Dent 2011;28(1):8–15.
76. Mullen HS, Scavelli TD, Quesenberry KE, et al. Gastrointestinal Foreign Body in Ferrets: 25 Cases (1986 to 1990). J Am Anim Hosp Assoc 1992;28(1):13–9.
77. Watson MK, Cazzini P, Mayer J, et al. Histology and immunohistochemistry of severe inflammatory bowel disease versus lymphoma in the ferret (Mustela putorius furo). J Vet Diagn Invest 2016;28(3):198–206.
78. Cazzini P, Watson MK, Gottdenker N, et al. Proposed grading scheme for inflammatory bowel disease in ferrets and correlation with clinical signs. J Vet Diagn Invest 2020;32(1):17–24.
79. Pollock C. Mycobacterial infection in the ferret. Vet Clin North Am Exot Anim Pract 2012;15(1):121–9.
80. Davendralingam N, Davagnanam I, Stidworthy MF, et al. Transmission of Mycobacterium xenopi to a pet albino ferret (Mustela putorius furo) from a domestic aquarium. Vet Rec 2017;181(7):169.
81. Dequeant B, Pascal Q, Bilbault H, et al. Identification of Mycobacterium genavense natural infection in a domestic ferret. J Vet Diagn Invest 2019;31(1):133–6.
82. Nakata M, Miwa Y, Tsuboi M, et al. Mycobacteriosis in a domestic ferret (Mustela putorius furo). J Vet Med Sci 2014;76(5):705–9.
83. De Lorenzi G, Kamphuisen K, Biscontini G, et al. Mycobacterium genavense Infection in a Domestic Ferret (Mustela putorius furo). Top Companion Anim Med 2018;33(4):119–21.
84. Bezos J, Álvarez-Carrión B, Rodriguez-Bertos A, et al. Evidence of disseminated infection by Mycobacterium avium subspecies hominissuis in a pet ferret (Mustela putorius furo). Res Vet Sci 2016;109(0):52–5.
85. Piseddu E, Trotta M, Tortoli E, et al. Detection and molecular characterization of Mycobacterium celatum as a cause of splenitis in a domestic ferret (Mustela putorius furo). J Comp Pathol 2011;144(2–3):214–8.
86. Lucas J, Lucas A, Furber H, et al. Mycobacterium genavense infection in two aged ferrets with conjunctival lesions. Aust Vet J 2000;78(10):685–9.
87. Morera N, Juan-Sallés C, Torres JM, et al. Cryptococcus gattii infection in a Spanish pet ferret (Mustela putorius furo) and asymptomatic carriage in ferrets and humans from its environment. Med Mycol 2011;49(7):779–84.
88. Malik R, Alderton B, Finlaison D, et al. Cryptococcosis in ferrets: a diverse spectrum of clinical disease. Aust Vet J 2002;80(12):749–55.
89. Miwa Y, Kurosawa A, Ogawa H, et al. Neoplasitic diseases in ferrets in Japan: a questionnaire study for 2000 to 2005. J Vet Med Sci 2009;71(4):397–402.
90. Avallone G, Forlani A, Tecilla M, et al. Neoplastic diseases in the domestic ferret (Mustela putorius furo) in Italy: classification and tissue distribution of 856 cases (2000-2010). BMC Vet Res 2016;12(1):275.
91. Shoemaker NJ, Schuurmans M, Moorman H, et al. Correlation between age at neutering and age at onset of hyperadrenocorticism in ferrets. J Am Vet Med Assoc 2000;216(2):195–7.
92. Li X, Fox JG, Padrid PA. Neoplastic diseases in ferrets: 574 cases (1968-1997). J Am Vet Med Assoc 1998;212(9):1402–6.

93. Rhody JL, Williams BH. Exocrine Pancreatic Adenocarcinoma and Associated Extrahepatic Biliary Obstruction in a Ferret. J Exot Pet Med 2013;22(2):206–11.
94. Suran JN, Wyre NR. Imaging Findings In 14 Domestic Ferrets (Mustela Putorius Furo) With Lymphoma. Vet Radiol Ultrasound 2011;0(0):1–10.
95. Onuma M, Kondo H, Ono S, et al. Cytomorphological and immunohistochemical features of lymphoma in ferrets. J Vet Med Sci 2008;70(9):893–8.
96. Erdman SE, Correa P, Coleman LA, et al. Helicobacter mustelae-associated gastric MALT lymphoma in ferrets. Am J Pathol 1997;151:273–80.
97. Hanley CS, Wilson GH, Frank P. T cell lymphoma in the lumbar spine of a domestic ferret (Mustela putorius furo). Vet Rec 2004;155:329–33.
98. Bean AD, Fisher PG, Reavill DR, et al. Hypercalcemia associated with lymphomas in the ferret (Mustela putorius furo): four cases. J Exot Pet Med 2019; 29:147–53.
99. Ammersbach M, DeLay J, Caswell JL, et al. Laboratory Findings, Histopathology, and Immunophenotype of Lymphoma in Domestic Ferrets. Vet Pathol 2008; 45(5):663–73.
100. Rosenbaum MR, Affolter VK, Usborne AL, et al. Cutaneous epitheliotropic lymphoma in a ferret. J Am Vet Med Assoc 1996;209(8):1441–4.
101. Vilalta L, Meléndez-Lazo A, Doria G, et al. Clinical, Cytological, Histological and Immunohistochemical Features of Cutaneous Mast Cell Tumours in Ferrets (Mustela putorius furo). J Comp Pathol 2014;155(4):346–55.
102. Mikaelian I, Garner MM. Solitary dermal leiomyosarcomas in 12 ferrets. J Vet Diagn Invest 2002;14(3):262–5.

Printed and bound by CPI Group (UK) Ltd, Croydon, CR0 4YY

03/10/2024

01040480-0003